Caring for Patients Across the Cancer Care Continuum

W0106345

Larissa Nekhlyudov
Mita Sanghavi Goel
Jenny J. Lin
Linda Overholser
Kimberly S. Peairs
Editors

Caring for Patients Across the Cancer Care Continuum

Essentials for Primary Care

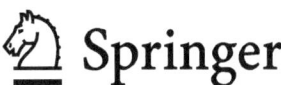 Springer

Editors
Larissa Nekhlyudov
Brigham and Women's Hospital
Harvard Medical School
Boston, MA
USA

Mita Sanghavi Goel
Feinberg School of Medicine
Northwestern University
Evanston, IL
USA

Jenny J. Lin
Icahn School of Medicine at
Mount Sinai
New York, NY
USA

Linda Overholser
University of Colorado School
of Medicine, Aurora
Aurora, CO
USA

Kimberly S. Peairs
Johns Hopkins School of
Medicine
Baltimore, MD
USA

ISBN 978-3-030-01895-5   ISBN 978-3-030-01896-2   (eBook)
https://doi.org/10.1007/978-3-030-01896-2

Library of Congress Control Number: 2018966805

This Springer imprint is published by the registered company Springer Nature Switzerland AG
The registered company address is: Gewerbestrasse 11, 6330 Cham, Switzerland

Contents

Abbreviations

ACP	Advance care planning
ACS	American Cancer Society
ADT	Androgen deprivation therapy
AFP	Alpha fetoprotein
ATLL	Adult T-cell lymphoma
BCG	Bacille Calmette-Guérin [vaccine]
BSE	Breast self-exam
CBE	Clinical breast exam
CRC	Colorectal cancer
DBT	Digital breast tomosynthesis
DES	Diethylstilbestrol
DM	Diagnostic mammography
DRE	Digital rectal exam
EBV	Epstein-Barr virus
ECOG	Eastern Cooperative Oncology Group
EGFR	Epidermal growth factor receptor
EUS	Endoscopic ultrasound
FNA	Fine-needle aspiration
GERD	Gastroesophageal reflux disease
GIST	Gastrointestinal stromal tumors
GVHD	Graft-versus-host disease
HBV	Hepatitis B virus
HCV	Hepatitis C virus
HPV	Human papillomavirus
HTLV-1	Human T-cell leukemia/lymphoma virus type 1
IARC	International Agency for Research on Cancer

IMRT	Intensity-modulated radiation therapy
KSVH	Kaposi sarcoma-associated herpesvirus
LDCT	Low-dose computed tomography
Mab	Monoclonal antibodies
MCPyV	Merkel cell polyomavirus
MDPOA	Medical durable power of attorney
MRCP	Magnetic resonance cholangiopancreatography
MRI	Magnetic resonance imaging
NAM	National Academy of Medicine
NHL	Non-Hodgkin lymphoma
NK	Natural killer [cells]
NLST	National Lung Screening Trial
NTP	National Toxicology Program
OIC	Opioid-induced constipation
PAD	Physician-assisted dying
PCP(s)	Primary care physician(s)
PD	Programmed death
PET (scan)	Positron emission tomography
POLST	Physician orders of life-sustaining treatment
PPV	Positive predictive value
SERM	Selective estrogen receptor modulator
SSRIs	Serotonin-specific reuptake inhibitors
TCAs	Tricyclic antidepressants
TKI	Tyrosine kinase inhibitors
TRUS	Transrectal ultrasound
USPSTF	United States Preventive Services Task Force
VEGF	Vascular endothelial growth factor [inhibitors]
YA	Young adult

Contributors

Mita Sanghavi Goel, MD, MPH Division of General Internal Medicine and Geriatrics, Feinberg School of Medicine, Northwestern University, Chicago, IL, USA

Jenny J. Lin, MD, MPH Division of General Internal Medicine, Icahn School of Medicine at Mount Sinai, New York, NY, USA

Larissa Nekhlyudov, MD, MPH Division of General Internal Medicine and Primary Care, Brigham and Women's Hospital, Harvard Medical School, Boston, MA, USA

Linda Overholser, MD Division of General Internal Medicine, University of Colorado School of Medicine, Aurora, CO, USA

Kimberly S. Peairs, MD Division of General Internal Medicine, Johns Hopkins University School of Medicine, Baltimore, MD, USA

Allison Wolfe, MD Division of General Internal Medicine, University of Colorado School of Medicine, Aurora, CO, USA

Chapter 1
Introduction and Overview

Larissa Nekhlyudov

Primary care providers can play a central or collaborative role in caring for patients newly diagnosed with cancer, cancer survivors, and those dying with cancer. In the United States, more than 1.7 million new cases of cancer are diagnosed each year and over 600,000 cancer deaths occur. As of 2016, there are over 15.5 million individuals who have survived or are living with cancer. It is estimated that by 2026, there will be 20.3 million cancer survivors. Among those newly diagnosed with cancer and those who are living with cancer, most are aged 65 and older and have comorbid medical conditions. While most patients diagnosed with cancer are older adults, cancer affecting younger populations may lead to a different set of challenges for survivors, namely, late and long-term effects of treatment causing significant morbidity and premature mortality.

Demand for cancer care is growing, driven by the rise in the incidence of the condition, earlier detection, increased survival, and the aging of the elderly population. Primary care providers play a critical role in the care of patients across the cancer continuum, from prevention to screening, diagnosis

L. Nekhlyudov (✉)
Division of General Internal Medicine and Primary Care,
Brigham and Women's Hospital, Harvard Medical School,
Boston, MA, USA
e-mail: lnekhlyudov@partners.org

© Springer Nature Switzerland AG 2019   1
L. Nekhlyudov et al. (eds.), *Caring for Patients Across the Cancer Care Continuum*,
https://doi.org/10.1007/978-3-030-01896-2_1

and treatment, and through survivorship and end of life. Evidence has shown that when primary care providers are involved in the care of individuals living with cancer, the quality of their care is more comprehensive; yet, many internists lack the confidence to care for this patient population. The *2013 Institute of Medicine* report advised that all providers caring for cancer patients across the continuum should have appropriate core competencies to do so. Across the cancer care trajectory, primary care providers interact with numerous specialists, thus communication and coordination are of vital importance (Fig. 1.1).

In this handbook, we aim to help primary care providers to offer high-quality care to patients by providing them with core competencies across the cancer care continuum. Each chapter is formatted as an outline, with the intention of serving as a place to find specific facts and recommendations quickly within more general topics. Specifically, the chapters include the following:

Prevention

- This chapter provides an overview of factors that contribute to the development of cancer, including diet, exercise, smoking, alcohol, and genetics. The chapter offers recommendations for counseling patients and how to incorporate prevention into daily practice.

Screening

- This chapter provides an overview of current screening guidelines, offers suggestions for patient engagement and decision-making, and addresses disparities in cancer screening.

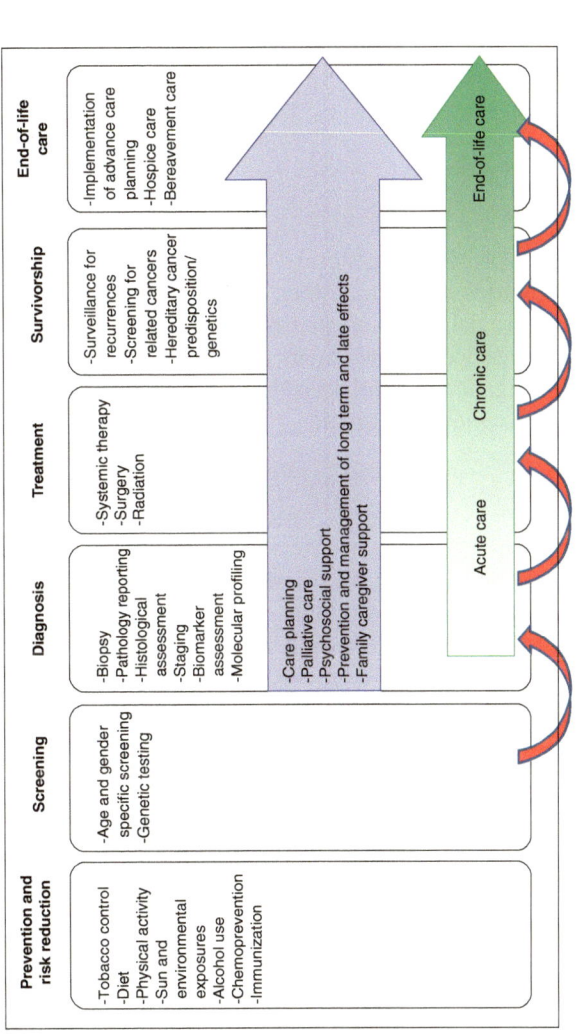

FIGURE. 1.1 Care transitions from primary to specialty care. (Modified and reprinted with permission from Delivering high-quality cancer care: charting a new course for a system in crisis, 2013, by the National Academy of Sciences, Courtesy of the National Academies Press, Washington, DC)

Diagnosis

- This chapter describes the epidemiology of cancer diagnoses, provides an overview of "alarm" symptoms that should trigger additional evaluation, and addresses disparities in cancer diagnosis.

Treatment

- This chapter provides a general overview of cancer treatment modalities and guidelines, including information about acute toxicities associated with treatment regimens and recommended management, and offers suggestions for patient engagement and decision-making, and addresses disparities in cancer treatment.

Survivorship

- This chapter provides an overview of cancer survivorship care focusing on those who have completed treatment. It offers recommendations for cancer surveillance, screening for other cancers, as well as surveillance and management of late physical and psychosocial effects. Health promotion, disease prevention, and care coordination are addressed.

Palliative/End-of-Life Care

- This chapter provides an overview of issues surrounding end-of-life care and management of symptoms. Insights are offered about communication, addressing goals of care, and strategies to assist in decision-making.

We hope that this handbook proves to be a go to guide for primary care providers as they care for patients across the cancer care continuum.

References

Bluethmann SM, Mariotto AB, Rowland JH. Anticipating the "Silver Tsunami": prevalence trajectories and comorbidity burden among older cancer survivors in the United States. Cancer Epidemiol Biomarkers Prev. 2016;25(7):1029–36.

IOM (Institute of Medicine). Delivering high-quality cancer care: charting a new course for a system in crisis. Washington, DC: The National Academies Press; 2013.

Miller KD, Siegel RL, Lin CC, Mariotto AB, Kramer JL, Rowland JH, et al. Cancer treatment and survivorship statistics, 2016. CA Cancer J Clin. 2016;66(4):271–89.

Siegel RL, Miller KD, Jemal A. Cancer statistics, 2018. CA Cancer J Clin. 2018;68(1):7–30.

Chapter 2
Cancer Prevention

Mita Sanghavi Goel and Linda Overholser

Overview

Cancer prevention refers to activities that help to reduce the incidence and overall burden of cancer. It can include screening, but more broadly encompasses other activities in the clinical setting as well as individual behaviors. Traditionally, prevention has been defined in tiers of primary, secondary, and tertiary prevention.

Definition of Prevention Terms

- *Primary Prevention:* Activities that help to reduce the risk of cancer ever developing

M. S. Goel (✉)
Division of General Internal Medicine and Geriatrics,
Feinberg School of Medicine, Northwestern University,
Chicago, IL, USA
e-mail: Mita.Goel@nm.org

L. Overholser
Division of General Internal Medicine, University of Colorado
School of Medicine, Aurora, CO, USA

© Springer Nature Switzerland AG 2019   7
L. Nekhlyudov et al. (eds.), *Caring for Patients Across the
Cancer Care Continuum*,
https://doi.org/10.1007/978-3-030-01896-2_2

- Counseling for modifiable behavioral risk factors known to influence the risk of cancer
- Vaccinations
- Genetic counseling/testing with recommendations for screening

- *Secondary Prevention:* Activities that detect and/or treat cancer at precancerous stages or at a stage before symptoms are present

  - Cancer screening tests (e.g., mammography, colonoscopy)
  - Surgery, chemotherapy, or radiation therapy

- *Tertiary Prevention:* Activities that aim to reduce the complications or recurrence of cancer

  - Screening for secondary cancers
  - Chemoprevention (e.g., tamoxifen for estrogen receptor-positive breast cancer)
  - Therapies to relieve symptoms
  - Counseling to improve quality of life
  - Surveillance for late effects of cancer and its treatment

As more individuals are living with a history of cancer and with a growing recognition of the late and long-term effects of cancer, these tiers may become difficult to distinguish.

Epidemiology of Risk Factors

- *Genetic risk factors.* Population-level prevalence of genetic risk factors is not readily available for most inherited mutations and may vary significantly between different populations. For example, the prevalence of BRCA 1 and 2 gene mutations is estimated at 1–2 in 1000 in the general population, compared with 1 in 100 among Ashkenazi Jews
- *Nongenetic risk factors.* In contrast, based on prevalence estimates of overweight and obesity alone, the majority of the adult US population has at least one nongenetic cancer risk factor

Genetic Risk Factors for Cancer

- Inherited genetic risk factors
  - Genetic mutations, or alterations in the makeup of an individual's DNA, can be present from birth (i.e., germ-line mutations) and are present in every cell of an individual
  - Contribute to about 5–10% of all cancer cases in the United States
  - Certain cancers occur in above-normal frequency or in clusters among blood relatives with regular patterns of inheritance and can be classified into known cancer syndromes. More than 50 of these hereditary cancer syndromes have been identified (Table 2.1)

- Acquired genetic risk factors

TABLE 2.1 Common genetic mutations increasing risk of cancer

Genetic mutation (syndrome)	Normal function of gene	Most common associated cancers
TP53 (Li-Fraumeni syndrome)	Produces protein that suppresses tumor growth	Breast Osteosarcoma Soft tissue sarcomas
BRCA 1/2	Produces protein that suppresses tumor growth	Breast Ovarian Pancreatic Prostate
PTN (Cowden syndrome)	Produces protein that suppresses tumor growth	Breast Thyroid Endometrial
MLH1, HSM 2, MSH6, PMS2, EPCAM (Lynch syndrome, hereditary nonpolyposis colorectal cancer)	Involved in repairing DNA damaged during replication	Colorectal Stomach, small intestine Liver Ovarian Uterine

- Occur from changes in the DNA that arise over time and are caused by errors during division of individual cells or by damage caused to DNA by external factors such as radiation (including UV radiation as in the case of melanoma)

Nongenetic Risk Factors for Cancer

Modifiable, Nongenetic Risk Factors

Comorbidities/Medical Exposures

- Inflammation

  - Conditions with chronic inflammation, such as Crohn's disease and ulcerative colitis, have increased risk of colorectal cancer

- Hormonal Exposure

  - Use of estrogen therapy alone in postmenopausal women increases risk of endometrial cancer
  - Combined estrogen and progestin likely increases risk of breast cancer
  - Endogenous hormonal production, especially estrogen production, appears to increase risk of breast cancer. As a result, some breast cancer risk calculators incorporate age of menarche and/or menopause, parity, and age at first full-term pregnancy
  - Diethylstilbestrol (DES) exposure. Women who took DES during pregnancy may have an increased risk of breast cancer. Daughters of these women have increased risk of cancers of the cervix and vagina

- Immunosuppression

  - *Organ transplant patients.* These patients are at increased risk of numerous cancers, especially non-Hodgkin's lymphoma (NHL), lung cancer, renal cancer, and liver cancer. This may be related to susceptibility to infections related to cancer: hepatitis B, hepatitis C, and Epstein-Barr virus (EBV), as well as susceptibility to cellular damage leading to development of lung and renal cancers

– *HIV*. These patients are at an increased risk of both infection-related and non-infection-related cancers. The primary non-infection-related cancer is lung cancer. Infection-related cancers include cancers associated with EBV (NHL), human herpesvirus-8 (Kaposi sarcoma-associated virus), hepatitis B and C viruses (liver cancers), and human papillomavirus (cervical, anal, oropharyngeal cancers)

- Infectious Agents

   – *Epstein-Barr Virus (EBV)*. Type of herpes virus that causes mononucleosis. Associated with certain types of lymphoma and oropharyngeal cancers

   – *Hepatitis B Virus (HBV)*. Chronic infection can cause liver cancer. Widespread immunization against hepatitis B began during the 1980s. HBV can be transmitted via blood, vertically from the mother to the infant at birth, and through sexual contact

   – *Hepatitis C Virus (HCV)*. Chronic infection associated with liver cancer. Universal screening for those born between 1945 and 1965 recommended

   – *HIV*. Per Immunosuppression section above

   – *Human Papillomavirus (HPV)*. Causes nearly all cervical cancers and most anal cancers. Also cause many oropharyngeal, vaginal, vulvar, and penile cancers. Vaccines have been developed for most cancer-causing HPV strains. Vaccination available for children as young as 9 years of age. Recommended for both boys and girls

   – *Human T-Cell Leukemia/Lymphoma Virus Type 1 (HTLV-1)*. Can cause adult T-cell lymphoma (ATLL), which is an aggressive type of non-Hodgkin's lymphoma found more commonly in Japan, Africa, the Caribbean, and South America. Spread through sexual contact, blood, or vertically from mothers to children while pregnant or breastfeeding

- *Kaposi Sarcoma-Associated Herpesvirus (KSVH), Also Known as Human herpesvirus-8.* Can cause Kaposi sarcoma, primary effusion lymphoma, and multicentric Castleman disease. Can be spread through saliva or organ or bone marrow transplantation, but patterns of transmission vary globally. In the United States and Northern Europe, it appears most commonly transmitted sexually, particularly among men who have sex with men
- *Merkel Cell Polyomavirus (MCPyV).* MCPyV can cause Merkel cell carcinoma, an uncommon form of skin cancer. The virus is most likely transmitted through skin-to-skin contact or through indirect contact (i.e., touching a surface previously touched by an infected person). More common among elderly and young adults with immunosuppression
- *Helicobacter pylori (H. pylori).* Causes noncardia gastric cancer and gastric MALT lymphoma, which affects the stomach lining. Thought to be spread by contaminated food or water and direct mouth-to-mouth contact, particularly in areas with crowding and poor sanitation. Infection is more common in Asia and South America than in the United States. Eradication of *H. pylori* as a prevention strategy is being studied
- *Opisthorchis viverrini.* A parasitic flatworm found in Southeast Asia that causes cholangiocarcinoma. Infection occurs by eating raw or undercooked freshwater fish containing larvae. Treated with antiparasitic medications
- *Schistosoma hematobium.* A parasitic flatworm found in freshwater snails in Africa and the Middle East and causes bladder cancer. Infection occurs when swimming in freshwater in contaminated areas

Lifestyle/Health Behaviors (Including Occupational Exposures)

- Alcohol Consumption
  - About 3.5% of all cancer deaths are considered alcohol related

– Associated with increased risk of:

  • Head and neck cancers: oral pharyngeal, and laryngeal cancers
  • Liver cancer
  • Squamous cell esophageal cancer
  • Colorectal cancer
  • Breast cancer

– May be associated with:

  • Renal cell carcinoma
  • Non-Hodgkin's lymphoma

– Increased risk related to amount of alcohol consumed daily. For example:

  • Head and neck cancer risk two- to threefold higher in those drinking 3.5 or more alcoholic drinks daily
  • Breast cancer risk increased by 7–12% per alcoholic drink (10 grams) consumed daily

– Concomitant tobacco use further increases risk of head and neck and esophageal cancers
– Certain enzymes (e.g., alcohol dehydrogenase and alcohol dehydrogenase 2) may further affect cancer risk. These enzymes can increase metabolism of alcohol to acetaldehyde and thus lead to higher risk of cancer among those with these enzymes who drink alcohol
– Potential mechanisms for carcinogenesis include:

  • DNA damage from buildup of metabolites, such as acetaldehyde
  • DNA damage from oxidation
  • Impairing ability to break down or absorb nutrients affecting cancer risk
  • Increased estrogen blood levels

– Not well studied, but appears that risk decreases for certain cancers after cessation of alcohol intake. May take 10–15 years to start seeing risk reduction

- Environmental Carcinogen Exposure
    - A *carcinogen* is any substance that is considered to be a cause of cancer; can be chemicals, infectious agents, or naturally occurring substances such as radiation. Substances listed in the National Toxicology Program (NTP) Report on carcinogens are classified using the following criteria:
        - *Known to be a human carcinogen*: Means that sufficient levels of evidence have been established to indicate a causal relationship between the substance and cancer in humans
        - *Reasonably anticipated to be a human carcinogen*: Means that:
            - The evidence to establish a causal relationship between the substance and human cancer is more limited, and other factors could explain the cancer.
            - The level of evidence is sufficient in animal studies, but the association has not established in humans
            - The level of evidence in both human and animal cancers is insufficient, but that similar structures have been listed previously in the NTP Report
    - Complete list of carcinogens compiled by the NTP is https://ntp.niehs.nih.gov/ntp/roc/content/listed_substances_508.pdf
    - International Agency for Research on Cancer (IARC), the cancer agency of the World Health Organization, list may be found at http://monographs.iarc.fr/ENG/Monographs/PDFs/index.php
- Diet
    - Most studies show associations with cancer, but are unable to prove causation
    - Foods or additives associated with increased risk of cancer:

- *Acrylamide*. Found in tobacco and certain foods, such as potatoes cooked at high temperature. Associated with increased cancer risk in animal models
- *Alcohol*. See above
- *Calcium*. May increase risk of prostate cancer and reduce risk of other cancers
- *Charred meat*, especially from muscle meat cooked at high temperature, creates chemicals (e.g., heterocyclic amines and polycyclic aromatic hydrocarbons) that are shown to cause cancer in animals

– Foods or additives associated with decreased risk of cancer:

- *Calcium*. Associated with decreased rate of colorectal cancer, but increased rate of prostate cancer
- *Cruciferous vegetables* (e.g., cauliflower, broccoli). Contain glucosinolates, which have certain breakdown products associated with cancer risk reduction
- *Garlic*. May reduce risk of gastrointestinal cancers

– Other foods and additives to consider:

- *Antioxidants*. Thought to decrease cancer risk by decreasing damage from some free radicals, but mixed results on reducing cancer risk among humans
- *Artificial sweeteners*. No conclusive evidence of increased cancer risk in artificial sweeteners sold in the United States, including saccharin, aspartame, and sucralose
- *Fluoride*. Found as additive to water, fluoride has not been shown to alter risk of cancer
- *Tea*. Contains certain antioxidants, but hasn't definitively shown cancer risk reduction
- *Vitamin D*. High intake may be associated with lower colorectal cancer risk; clinical trials are currently underway

- Obesity
  - Background
    - Most evidence comes from cohort studies, and describes associations, not causation. Thus, it is unclear if observed increase in risk is related to increased body fat or differences in lifestyle related to physical activity and diet
    - Obesity may be responsible for an estimated 28,000 new cases of cancer in 2012
  - Possible mechanisms altering cancer risk include:
    - Obesity may lead to an increased level of chronic inflammation or have obesity-associated conditions that increase chronic inflammation
    - Excess estrogen production from adipose tissue can lead to higher risk of cancer
    - Increased levels of insulin and insulin-like growth factor, which may increase risk of colon, endometrial, kidney, and prostate cancers
    - Altered levels of fat cell-associated hormones that stimulate and inhibit cell growth
    - Fat cells may affect other cell growth regulators, thus promoting cancer growth or reducing suppression
  - Effects of obesity on specific cancers:
    - *Breast cancer.* In postmenopausal women who never used hormone replacement, increased risk of hormone receptor-positive tumors. Decreased risk of hormone receptor-positive breast cancer among pre-menopausal overweight and obese women
    - *Colorectal cancer.* Slight increase in risk among obese individuals, especially men
    - *Endometrial cancer.* Two to four times more likely to occur in obese and overweight women. Appears to have increasing risk with increasing weight gain
    - *Esophageal adenocarcinoma.* Twice as likely among overweight and obese individuals

- *Gallbladder cancer.* Twenty percent increased risk among overweight and 60% increased risk among obese, especially among women
- *Gastric cardia cancer.* Almost twice as likely to occur among obese individuals
- *Liver cancer.* About twice as likely among obese and overweight individuals. This association appears stronger in men than women
- *Multiple myeloma.* Slightly increased risk among overweight and obese individuals
- *Meningioma.* About 50% increase in risk of developing among obese individuals
- *Ovarian cancer.* Increased risk among those women who never used hormone replacement therapy
- *Pancreatic cancer.* About 1.5 times more likely to develop in obese individuals
- *Renal cell cancer.* Almost twice as likely among overweight and obese individuals, even independent of hypertension
- *Thyroid cancer.* Slight increase in risk for every 5-point increase in BMI

- Radiation Exposures

  - Certain types of radiation, such as radon, X-rays, and gamma rays, are considered ionizing. This means it has enough energy to damage DNA and increase risk of cancer
  - Radon

    - Radioactive gas produced by soil and rocks
    - May be found in unventilated homes and basements in areas that have high levels of radon in the soil
    - Increases risk of lung cancer

  - High-energy radiation

    - Includes X-rays, gamma rays, alpha particles, beta particles, and neutrons
    - Associated with certain procedures, including X-rays, CT scans, positron emission tomography (PET) scans

- One regular dose CT scan is equivalent to 2 years of exposure to background radiation
- Associated with cancer treatment, such as mantle radiation for Hodgkin's lymphoma

- Ultraviolet Radiation

  - Found in natural sunlight, tanning beds, and sunlamps
  - Increase risk of skin cancers

- Tobacco

  - Leading cause of cancer and death from cancer
  - Increased risk for cancers of the larynx, lung, mouth, esophagus, throat, bladder, kidney, liver, stomach, pancreas, rectum, cervix, and acute myeloid leukemia
  - Smokeless tobacco increases risk of cancers of the mouth, esophagus, and pancreas

Non-modifiable, Nongenetic Risk Factors

- Age

  - Median age at cancer diagnosis is 66
  - Increasing age is associated with increasing incidence of cancer as seen in Fig. 2.1, though certain cancers (e.g., neuroblastomas) are more common at younger ages
  - Recalling link between age and cancer epidemiology can guide screening and diagnostic evaluations

Common Myths About Cancer Risk

- *Sugar*. Sugar has not been directly linked to increased risk of cancer, independent of its relationship to obesity
- *Artificial sweeteners*. No consistent link between aspartame, saccharin, sucralose, and cancer has been identified
- *Cell phones*. Cell phones emit a low-frequency energy that does not appear to damage cells, and no definitive association has been found

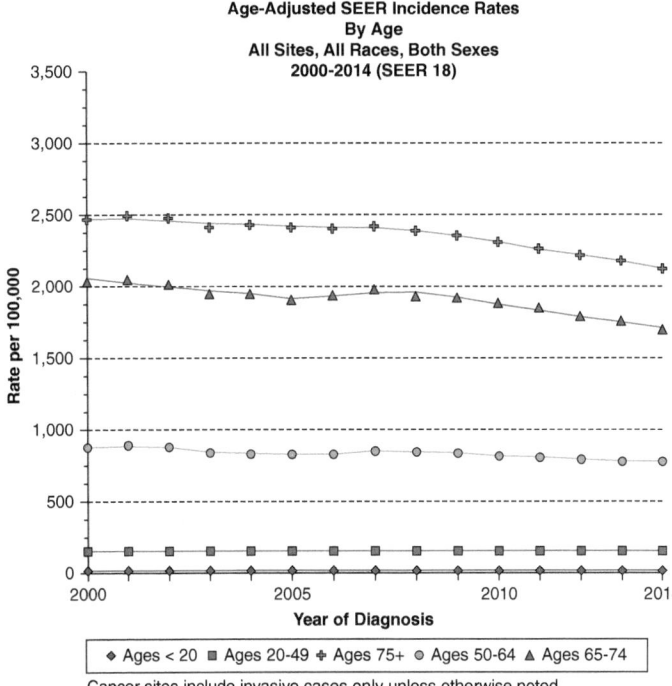

FIGURE 2.1 Cancer incidence by age. Figure generated using software from Fast Stats: An interactive tool for access to SEER cancer statistics. Surveillance Epidemiology and End Results *(SEER)* Program, National Cancer Institute. https://seer.cancer.gov/faststats

- *Power lines.* Power lines emit both electrical and magnetic energy. Electrical energy is typically blocked by walls, and magnetic energy is a low-frequency energy that does not lead to DNA damage
- *Nutritional supplements.* No supplements have yet been shown to reduce risk of any type of cancer, with the exception of calcium for prostate cancer

  - Use of beta-carotene and vitamin E may have more risks than benefits, and use should be discouraged for cancer prevention

- *Deodorant and antiperspirant.* No increased risk of cancer seen among those using deodorant and antiperspirant
- *Hair dye.* There is no link between personal hair dye use and cancer, though professionals in contact with hair dye have increased risk of developing bladder cancer

Role of Primary Care in Prevention

The primary care provider has an important role to play in identifying important risk factors, counseling individuals on health behaviors, and initiating screening or other strategies that can help reduce the risk for cancer or detect cancer at earlier, more favorable stages. Specific strategies to modify the risk of cancer include:

- Address and mitigate modifiable risk factors from the list above, including diet and exercise
    - Provide *risk-based care* for individuals whose risk may be elevated due to hereditary syndromes or previous cancer treatments
        - Appropriately modify screening if deemed at increased risk
        - Consider referral for genetic counseling and possible testing if hereditary component is suspected
- Detect precancerous conditions early (e.g., identify and remove adenomatous polyp during screening colonoscopy) *(see also* Chap. 3*)*
- Discuss chemoprevention—use of a medication to lower risk of developing cancer
    - Selective estrogen receptor modulators, such as tamoxifen, lower risk of breast cancer in high-risk women
    - Finasteride lowers risk of prostate cancer
    - COX-2 inhibitors may prevent colon and breast cancer
    - Aspirin may prevent colon cancer

- Refer for elective surgery
  - Prophylactic bilateral mastectomy
  - Risk-reducing salpingo-oophorectomy
  - Hysterectomy and bilateral salpingo-oophorectomy
  - Colectomy for high-risk conditions, such as HNPCC or long-standing inflammatory bowel disease

Identifying and Counseling for Acquired or Modifiable Risk Factors

Risk factors that are potentially modifiable by lifestyle intervention account for approximately 40% of adult cancers. These and other acquired risk factors can be assessed with a thorough review of:

- *Past medical history.* For example, relevant infections or immune-related conditions, past cancer, or treatment exposures that could impact future cancer risk, vaccination status, history of hormone use, pregnancy, and comorbidities associated with cancer risk
- *Social history.* Determine smoking status, level of alcohol use, relevant sexual history, and occupational and recreational exposures. Includes evaluating health behaviors such as dietary and physical activity habits, use of tanning beds, use of supplements, etc
- *Family history.* Identifying patterns that suggest hereditary cancer syndromes
- *Medications.* For example, hormonal therapy or immune-suppressive regimens may lead to increased risk of certain cancers (Table 2.2)

Counseling for healthy lifestyle should be provided regularly:

- The five A's approach has been shown to be effective (*A*ssess, *A*dvise, *A*gree, *A*ssist, *A*rrange)
- Smoking cessation counseling for patients may also be available through lung cancer screening programs
- Motivational interviewing is helpful to identify and address barriers to behavior change

TABLE 2.2 Identifying and counseling for cancer risk factors

Timing during exam	Items pertinent to cancer prevention	Examples to identify pertinent to cancer prevention	Actionable recommendation
Past medical/ surgical history	Comorbid conditions	Ulcerative colitis	Identification
	Therapies that increase risk for cancer	Organ transplantation	Obtaining treatment information/records
		Infections (i.e., *H. pylori*; hepatitis B, C; HPV; HIV)	Confirming diagnostic/ treatment details
		Previous cancer	Modification of screening if appropriate
		Previous radiation therapy/bone marrow transplant	
Medications		Steroids	Identification and confirmation
		Immune-modulating agents	Counseling
		Immune suppressive therapies	Discontinuation if appropriate
		Hormone use	
		Supplement use	

| Family history | Third-generation family pedigree | Cancer diagnosis
Age at diagnosis
Ethnicity of individual
Associated medical conditions
Results of any previous genetic testing | Identification
Referral for genetic counseling/testing
Modification of screening if appropriate |
| Social history | Occupational, recreational exposures
Health behaviors | Exposure to asbestos, sun, radiation, harmful chemicals
Diet/nutrition (including use of supplements)
Exercise patterns
Sexual history
Birth history
Smoking/tobacco use
Use of sunscreen/tanning beds | Assessment
Counseling to reduce risk
Referrals if appropriate |

Dietary and physical activity guidelines for cancer prevention are updated at regular intervals by the American Cancer
Society. Current recommendations are included in Table 2.3.

Soliciting an Adequate Family History and Recognizing Hereditary Cancer Syndromes

It is important to obtain enough information about the family
history to be useful for the purposes of assessing hereditary
risk. A three-generation family history should be the ideal
goal:

- *First-degree relative*: Includes biological parents, siblings,
  and children
- *Second-degree relative*: Includes biological grandparents,
  aunts, uncles, nieces, nephews, and half-siblings
- *Third-degree relative*: Includes biological first cousins,
  great-grandparents, or great-grandchildren

(a) Family history should be obtained during a comprehen-
    sive review of history even before a cancer diagnosis is
    considered and should be updated at regular intervals,
    since family history may change over time
(b) Information to include for each individual ideally includes
    diagnosis, age at diagnosis, and ethnicity, if known
(c) Examples of factors that suggest a hereditary predisposi-
    tion to cancer for some common/more prevalent cancers
    include (adapted with permission from Hampel et al,
    2014):

    - *Breast cancer:*

        - Premenopausal breast cancer
        - Bilateral breast cancer in one individual
        - Triple negative breast cancer ≤ 60 years of age
        - Breast cancer in any male family member
        - ≥ 3 family members with history of breast, ovarian,
          pancreatic, or aggressive prostate cancer
        - Ashkenazi Jewish ethnicity

TABLE 2.3 Dietary and physical activity guidelines

Achieve and maintain a healthy weight throughout life

Be as lean as possible throughout life without being underweight

Avoid excess weight gain at all ages. For those who are currently overweight or obese, losing even a small amount of weight has health benefits and is a good place to start

Engage in regular physical activity and limit consumption of high-calorie foods and beverages as key strategies for maintaining a healthy weight

Adopt a physically active lifestyle

Adults should engage in at least 150 min of moderate intensity or 75 min of vigorous intensity activity each week, or an equivalent combination, preferably spread throughout the week

Children and adolescents should engage in at least 1 h of moderate or vigorous intensity activity each day, with vigorous intensity activity occurring at least 3 days each week

Limit sedentary behavior such as sitting, lying down, watching television, or other forms of screen-based entertainment

Doing some physical activity above usual activities, no matter what one's level of activity, can have many health benefits

Consume a healthy diet, with an emphasis on plant foods

Choose foods and beverages in amounts that help achieve and maintain a healthy weight

Limit consumption of processed meat and red meat

Eat at least 2.5 cups of vegetables and fruits each day

Choose whole grains instead of refined grain products

If you drink alcoholic beverages, limit consumption

Drink no more than 1 drink per day for women or 2 per day for men

From Kushi LH, Doyle C, McCullough M, et al. American Cancer Society guidelines on nutrition and physical activity for cancer prevention. CA Cancer J Clin. 2012 62(1):30–67. Used with permission from John Wiley & Sons

- History of breast cancer and any of the following cancers in the same individual or in two relatives, one of whom was diagnosed under the age of 45:
  - Soft tissue sarcoma
  - Osteosarcoma
  - Brain tumor
  - Adrenocortical tumor
  - Leukemia
  - Bronchoalveolar cancer
  - Colorectal cancer

- Personal history of breast cancer and ≥ 1 Peutz-Jeghers GI polyp
- Personal history of both lobular breast cancer and diffuse gastric cancer OR history of two relatives with each cancer, one of which diagnosed under the age of 50
- Personal history of both breast cancer and two additional criteria for Cowden syndrome

- Basal cell skin cancer:

  - >5 cumulative basal cell cancers in the same individual
  - Basal cell cancer under age 30 with one other criteria for nevoid basal cell carcinoma syndrome in the same individual

- Colorectal cancer:

  - Personal diagnosis under the age of 50
  - Personal diagnosis over the age of 50 with first-degree relative with either endometrial or colorectal cancer at any age
  - Personal history of synchronous or metachronous colorectal and/or endometrial cancer
  - Colorectal cancer with evidence of mismatch repair deficiency on tumor screen

- Colorectal cancer with history of ≥10 cumulative adenomatous polyps
- History of colorectal cancer and any of the following cancers in the same individual or in two relatives, one of whom was diagnosed under the age of 45:

  - Soft tissue sarcoma
  - Osteosarcoma
  - Brain tumor
  - Breast cancer
  - Adrenocortical tumor
  - Leukemia
  - Bronchoalveolar cancer

- Personal history of colorectal cancer and two additional Cowden syndrome criteria
- In the same individual or in close relatives, colorectal cancer and two of the following additional cancers:

  - Endometrial adenocarcinoma
  - Urothelial carcinoma
  - Gastric cancer
  - Ovarian cancer
  - Small bowel cancer
  - Glioblastoma
  - Sebaceous adenocarcinoma
  - Biliary tract cancer
  - Pancreatic cancer

- *Endometrial cancer*:

  - Diagnosis under the age of 50
  - Diagnosis over the age of 50 if any first-degree relative with history of colorectal or endometrial cancer
  - Synchronous or metachronous colorectal or endometrial cancer in the same individual
  - Evidence of mismatch repair deficiency on tumor screening

- In the same individual or in close relatives, endometrial cancer and two of the following additional cancers:

    – Colorectal cancer
    – Urothelial carcinoma
    – Gastric cancer
    – Ovarian cancer
    – Small bowel cancer
    – Glioblastoma
    – Sebaceous adenocarcinoma
    – Biliary tract cancer
    – Pancreatic cancer

  - Personal history of epithelial endometrial cancer and two additional Cowden syndrome criteria

- *Ovarian cancer:*

  - Any history of ovarian, primary peritoneal, or fallopian tube cancer in patient or first-degree relative

- *Malignant melanoma:*

  - ≥3 cases of melanoma and/or pancreatic cancer in patient or close relatives
  - ≥3 primary melanomas in the same individual
  - Melanoma and pancreatic cancer in the same individual
  - Melanoma and astrocytoma in the same individual or in first-degree relatives

- *Leukemia:*

  - Diagnosis <age 18 if any of the following present:

    – Consanguineous parents
    – Any second primary cancer
    – Sibling with childhood cancer
    – Café au lait macules or other signs of neurofibromatosis type 1
    – Family history of Lynch syndrome-associated cancers

- Leukemia and one other of the following cancers, in the same individual or in close relatives, one of whom is ≤45 years old:
    - Soft tissue sarcoma
    - Osteosarcoma
    - Brain tumor
    - Breast cancer
    - Adrenocortical cancer
    - Bronchoalveolar cancer
    - Colorectal cancer

- *Prostate cancer*:
    - ≥2 cases of prostate cancer under the age of 55 in close relatives
    - ≥3 first-degree relatives with prostate cancer
    - Aggressive (higher than Gleason score 7) prostate cancer with ≥2 cases of breast, ovarian, and/or pancreatic cancer in close relatives

Facilitating Referrals for Individuals Who May Be at Increased Risk for Cancer

- For individuals suspected of being at elevated risk of cancer based on family history or based on characteristics of a diagnosed cancer, referral for *genetics consultation* is appropriate

    - For consideration of BRCA risk assessment, use of specific tools designed for this purpose (as opposed to general risk assessment tools based on the Gail Model) is recommended by the US Preventive Services Task Force. Examples of tools include:

        - Ontario Risk Assessment Tool
        - Manchester Scoring System
        - Referral Screening Tool
        - Pedigree Assessment Tool
        - Family History Screen 7 (FHS-7)

- Consultation should include counseling and a thorough review of the patient family pedigree and clinical characteristics
- Referral for consultation does not guarantee that testing will be done
- If genetic testing is deemed appropriate, then both pre- and posttest counseling should be provided, along with interpretation of results and recommendations for surveillance
- See the *Additional Resources* below for sites to search for genetic counselors if uncertain about resources in your area

- High-risk cancer clinics may assist in making recommendations for chemoprevention
- Wellness programs, nutritional counseling, and/or referral for bariatric surgery may be helpful if available
- Surgery may be appropriate as a risk-reduction strategy in certain high-risk individuals:

  - Bilateral prophylactic mastectomy can reduce risk and may be considered in women with BRCA1/2 or other mutations that increase risk of breast cancer (i.e., TP53), a very strong family history, or a lifetime risk of breast cancer over 20%
  - Risk-reducing salpingo-oophorectomy can reduce risk for breast and ovarian cancer for women with BRCA1/2 mutations

    - Ideally should be performed after childbearing is complete in shared decision-making with the patient

  - Hysterectomy and bilateral salpingo-oophorectomy could be considered to reduce risk of endometrial and ovarian cancer in women with hereditary nonpolyposis colon cancer
  - Prophylactic colectomy may be considered to reduce risk for colon cancer:

- In individuals with long-standing (>10 years) ulcerative colitis (UC)
- In individuals with UC with dysplastic polyps on surveillance colonoscopy
- In individuals with familial adenomatous polyposis who have multiple polyps, dysplastic polyps, an increasing number of polyps on surveillance colonoscopy or who are unable to complete surveillance screening

Additional Resources

- Risk Calculators

  - Breast (B-RST): https://www.breastcancergenescreen.org/
  - Colorectal Cancer Risk Assessment Tool (NCI): https://www.cancer.gov/colorectalcancerrisk/

- List of Carcinogens

  - NTP: https://ntp.niehs.nih.gov/ntp/roc/content/listed_substances_508.pdf
  - International Agency for Research on Cancer (IARC), the cancer agency of the World Health Organization, list may be found at http://monographs.iarc.fr/ENG/Monographs/PDFs/index.php

- National Comprehensive Cancer Network: https://www.nccn.org/ (available with free registration)
- American Cancer Society: https://www.cancer.org/
- National Cancer Institute: https://www.cancer.gov/
- National Cancer Institute Cancer Genetics Services Directory: http://www.cancer.gov/cancertopics/genetics/directory
- National Society of Genetic Counselors: http://www.nsgc.org/
- American College of Genetics and Genomics: http://www.acmg.net/

References

Ashton-Prolla P, Giacomazzi J, Schmidt AV, Roth FL, Palmero EI, Kalakun L, et al. Development and validation of a simple questionnaire for the identification of hereditary breast cancer in primary care. BMC Cancer. 2009;9:283.

Baan R, Straif K, Grosse Y, Secretan B, El Ghissassi F, Bouvard V, et al. Carcinogenicity of alcoholic beverages. Lancet Oncol. 2007;8(4):292–3.

Evans DG, Eccles DM, Rahman N, Young K, Bulman M, Amir E, et al. A new scoring system for the chances of identifying a BRCA1/2 mutation outperforms existing models including BRCAPRO. J Med Genet. 2004;41(6):474–80.

Fletcher RH, Fletcher SW, Fletcher GS. Clinical epidemiology: the essentials. Philadelphia: Wolters Kluwer Health/Lippincott Williams & Wilkins; 2012.

Gilpin CA, Carson N, Hunter AG. A preliminary validation of a family history assessment form to select women at risk for breast or ovarian cancer for referral to a genetics center. Clin Genet. 2000;58(4):299–308.

Hampel H, Bennett RL, Buchanan A, Pearlman R, Wiesner GL. A practice guideline from the American College of Medical Genetics and Genomics and the National Society of Genetic Counselors: referral indications for cancer predisposition assessment. Genet Med. 2014;17:70.

Hoskins KF, Zwaagstra A, Ranz M. Validation of a tool for identifying women at high risk for hereditary breast cancer in population-based screening. Cancer. 2006;107(8):1769–76.

IARC Helicobacter pylori Working Group. Helicobacter pylori eradication as a strategy for preventing gastric cancer. (IARC Working Group Reports, No. 8). Lyon, France: International Agency for Research on Cancer; 2014b2014a. http://www.iarc.fr/en/publications/pdfs-online/wrk/wrk8/index.php.

Islami F, Goding Sauer A, Miller KD, Siegel RL, Fedewa SA, Jacobs EJ, et al. Proportion and number of cancer cases and deaths attributable to potentially modifiable risk factors in the United States. CA Cancer J Clin. 2018;68(1):31–54.

Kushi LH, Doyle C, McCullough M, Rock CL, Demark-Wahnefried W, Bandera EV, et al. American Cancer Society guidelines on nutrition and physical activity for cancer prevention: reducing the risk of cancer with healthy food choices and physical activity. CA Cancer J Clin. 2012;62(1):30–67.

Lim U, Subar AF, Mouw T, Hartge P, Morton LM, Stolzenberg-Solomon R, et al. Consumption of aspartame-containing beverages and incidence of hematopoietic and brain malignancies. Cancer Epidemiol Biomark Prev. 2006;15(9):1654–9.

Lum A, Le Marchand L. A simple mouthwash method for obtaining genomic DNA in molecular epidemiological studies. Cancer Epidemiol Biomark Prev. 1998;7(8):719–24.

Moyer VA. Vitamin, mineral, and multivitamin supplements for the primary prevention of cardiovascular disease and cancer: U.S. Preventive services Task Force recommendation statement. Ann Intern Med. 2014a;160(8):558–64.

Moyer VA, on behalf of the USPSTF. Risk assessment, genetic counseling, and genetic testing for BRCA-related cancer in women: U.S. preventive services task force recommendation statement. Ann Intern Med. 2014b;160(4):271–81.

Nelson DE, Jarman DW, Rehm J, Greenfield TK, Rey G, Kerr WC, et al. Alcohol-attributable cancer deaths and years of potential life lost in the United States. Am J Pub Health. 2013;103(4):641–8.

NTP (National Toxicology Program). Report on carcinogens, fourteenth edition. Research Triangle Park: U.S. Department of Health and Human Services; 2016.

Pilarski R, Burt R, Kohlman W, Pho L, Shannon KM, Swisher E. Cowden syndrome and the PTEN hamartoma tumor syndrome: systematic review and revised diagnostic criteria. J Natl Cancer Inst. 2013;105(21):1607–16.

Piñeiro B, Simmons VN, Palmer AM, Correa JB, Brandon TH. Smoking cessation interventions within the context of low-dose computed tomography lung cancer screening: a systematic review. Lung Cancer. 2016;98:91–8.

Whittemore AS, Gong G, John EM, McGuire V, Li FP, Ostrow KL, et al. Prevalence of BRCA1 mutation carriers among U.S. non-Hispanic whites. Cancer Epidemiol Biomark Prev. 2004;13(12):2078–83.

Chapter 3
Cancer Screening

Mita Sanghavi Goel and Jenny J. Lin

Overview

Screening is a process of testing asymptomatic individuals. In 1968, the World Health Organization proposed a set of criteria to evaluate various screening tests, commonly known as "Wilson's criteria." In 2008, with acknowledgement of emerging criteria, the criteria were updated (Box 3.1). In this chapter, we consider a variety of screening strategies for the early detection of cancer. There are specific concepts related to screening that will be discussed.

M. S. Goel (✉)
Division of General Internal Medicine and Geriatrics, Feinberg School of Medicine, Northwestern University, Chicago, IL, USA
e-mail: Mita.Goel@nm.org

J. J. Lin
Division of General Internal Medicine, Icahn School of Medicine at Mount Sinai, New York, NY, USA

© Springer Nature Switzerland AG 2019   35
L. Nekhlyudov et al. (eds.), *Caring for Patients Across the Cancer Care Continuum*,
https://doi.org/10.1007/978-3-030-01896-2_3

Box 3.1 World Health Organization Screening Criteria

- The screening program should respond to a recognized need
- The objectives of screening should be defined at the outset
- There should be a defined population
- There should be scientific evidence of screening program effectiveness
- The program should integrate education, testing, clinical services, and program management
- There should be quality assurance, with mechanisms to minimize potential risks of screening
- The program should ensure informed choice, confidentiality, and respect for autonomy
- The program should promote equity and access to screening for the entire target population
- Program evaluation should be planned from the outset
- The overall benefits of screening should outweigh the harms

Reprinted from Andermann A, Blancquaert I, Beauchamp S, Dery V. Revisiting Wilson and Jungner in the genomic age: a review of screening criteria over the past 40 years. *Bull World Health Organ*. 2008;86(4): 317–319. Used with permission

Definitions

- True positive (TP): those who test positive with a test *and* have the disease in question
- True negative (TN): those without the disease in question who test negative

- False positive (FP): those who test positive *and* do not have the disease in question
- False negative (FN): those who test negative but *do* have the disease in question
- Sensitivity: determines the proportion of individuals with a specific condition that are identified by the test. It is statistically calculated as TP/disease positive
- Specificity: determines the proportion of individuals without disease who correctly test negative. It is calculated as TN/disease negative
- Overdiagnosis: diagnosis of a disease that would not have manifested clinically or caused harm during the individual's expected lifetime

Guideline Development and Implications on Cancer Screening Recommendations

- In 2011, the Institute of Medicine, now known as the National Academy of Medicine (NAM), acknowledged the proliferation of guidelines proposed to assist with clinical decision-making. Given the potential for heterogeneity in the rigor of guideline development processes, the IOM proposed a set of criteria for developing "rigorous, trustworthy" clinical practice guidelines. They proposed that trustworthy guidelines require attention to the following eight standards throughout the entire process of guideline development:

  - Establishing transparency
  - Management of conflict of interest
  - Guideline development group composition
  - Clinical practice guideline and systematic review intersection
  - Establishing evidence foundations for and rating strength of recommendations
  - Articulation of recommendations

- External review
- Updating

- This chapter presents a variety of different proposed guidelines, though not all have been recognized as following the process proposed by NAM. Of the clinical guidelines presented, the US Preventive Services Task Force (USPSTF) and the American Cancer Society (ACS) have been consistently cited as following best practices. We have also included other influential professional organizations that propose screening guidelines for clinicians involved in clinical care. Evidence is continuously being monitored, and organizations may change guidelines; thus primary care providers should check recommendations regularly to ensure they are current
- Strength of recommendations:

  - USPSTF grades its recommendations along two dimensions, the strength of evidence and magnitude of benefit (Table 3.1)
  - ACS dichotomizes recommendations into two broad grades that take into consideration both risks and benefits:

    - Strong recommendation: consensus that the benefits of adherence to the intervention outweigh the undesirable effects
    - Qualified recommendation: clear evidence of benefit of adherence to the intervention but less certainty

TABLE 3.1 USPSTF evidence grading criteria

| Certainty of net benefit | Magnitude of net benefit | | | |
	Substantial	Moderate	Small	Zero/ negative
High	A	B	C	D
Moderate	B	B	C	D
Low	Insufficient (I)			

about either the balance of benefits and harms or about patients' values and preferences, which could lead to different decisions

- Canadian Task Force (CTFPHC) assesses its recommendations along similar dimensions, but does not provide a specific grade

  • Strength of recommendation:

    - Strong: most people would want to follow the recommended course of action
    - Weak: most people would want to follow the recommended course of action, but many would not. Decision aids may be helpful in this situation

  • Quality of evidence:

    - High: highly confident that the true effect lies close to the estimated effect
    - Moderate: the true effect is likely to lie close to the estimated effect
    - Weak: the true effect may be substantially different from the estimated effect

• *Breast Cancer Screening*

  - Epidemiology

    • Estimated 250,000 women diagnosed with breast cancer annually in the USA
    • As of 2014, 3,327,552 women living with breast cancer
    • Estimated over 40,000 deaths annually

  - Benefits and harms of screening

    • Estimates of mortality reduction (i.e., benefit) and harms vary depending on age of initiation, screening interval, and data source evaluating mortality reduction
    • A detailed discussion of the various benefits and harms studies is beyond the scope of this handbook;

however, we highlight a few analyses from organizations that conducted systematic reviews of benefits and harms *and* followed processes deemed high quality by NAM

- Benefits

  - The primary intended benefit of screening is to detect breast cancer as early as possible, thereby reducing breast cancer-related morbidity and mortality
  - According to USPSTF analyses, for every 1000 women followed through their lifetimes:

    - Twenty-five women would die of breast cancer without screening
    - Eighteen women would die of breast cancer if they initiate screening every 2 years starting at age 50
    - Seventeen women would die of breast cancer if they initiate screening every 2 years starting at age 40

  - According to ACS analyses, screening reduced breast cancer mortality by 20% for all women of average risk

- Harms

  - The USPSTF quantifies risk of harms by providing estimates for 10,000 women aged 50 years or greater followed for 10 years and screened every 2 years. With this denominator, they reported 302 women would be diagnosed with breast cancer, 10 women would avoid breast cancer death with mammography, 173 would survive breast cancer regardless of screening, and 62 women would die of breast cancer regardless of screening. Additional harms include short-term anxiety and pain associated with testing, particularly abnormal testing. Cumulative radiation exposure appears to be low under typical screening conditions; therefore we do not discuss it in greater detail in this chapter. Adverse outcomes included:

- False-positive mammograms: 6130
- Negative biopsy: 940
- Overdiagnosis: 57

– Screening guidelines for screening women with average risk of breast cancer (Table 3.2)

- ACOG: American College of Gynecology
- AAFP: American Academy of Family Practice
- ACP: American College of Physicians
- ACR: American College of Radiology

– Special populations

- Screening recommendations apply to women at average risk of breast cancer
- Clinicians need to identify women considered high risk, as they may require additional screening (i.e., genetic counseling or testing, MRI screening) or prophylactic treatment (i.e., bilateral prophylactic mastectomy, chemoprevention)
- High-risk groups consist of:

  – Women with personal or family history of breast cancer
  – Personal history of ductal carcinoma in situ, lobular carcinoma in situ, atypical ductal hyperplasia, and atypical lobular hyperplasia
  – Known BRCA gene mutation
  – History of chest radiation between ages 10–30

- Have first-degree family members with, or personal history of, other hereditary syndromes associated with increased breast cancer risk (i.e., Li-Fraumeni syndrome, Cowden syndrome, Bannayan-Riley-Ruvalcaba syndrome)

Table 3.2 Breast cancer screening recommendations (current as of May 2018)

Organization	Age to start screening	Age to end screening	Mammogram	Clinical breast exam (CBE)	Breast self-exam (BSE)
USPSTF	40–49: individualized discussion (Grade C) 50: routinely recommended (Grade B)	75 and older: insufficient evidence to recommend for or against screening (Grade I)	40–49: every 2 years, if opts for screening (Grade C) 50–74: every 2 years (Grade B)	Insufficient evidence to recommend for or against CBE (Grade I)	Recommends *against* BSE (Grade D)
ACS	40–44: individualized discussion (qualified recommendation) 45: routinely recommended (strong recommendation)	75 and older: continue screening as long as health is good AND life expectancy is 10 years or longer	40–44: every year, if opts for screening (qualified recommendation) 45–54: every year (qualified recommendation) 55–74: every 2 years with option of annual (qualified recommendation)	Does not recommend CBE (qualified recommendation)	No recommendation for performance of, or instruction in, BSE

ACOG	40–49: offer screening using shared decision-making 50: initiate routine screening	75 and older: use shared decision-making to guide decision, informed by health status and longevity	Every 1–2 years after having shared decision-making discussion	25–39: may be offered every 1–3 years 40 years and older: may offer annually	Not recommended
AAFP or ACP	Mirror USPSTF				
ACR	40: routinely recommend	As long as life expectancy is $\geq$5–7 years based on age and health status	Every year	n/a	n/a

(continued)

TABLE 3.2 (continued)

Organization	Age to start screening	Age to end screening	Mammogram	Clinical breast exam (CBE)	Breast self-exam (BSE)
NCCN	40: routinely recommended		Every year	40 years and older: annual clinical encounter	n/a
Canadian Task Force on Preventive Health	40–49: recommend *not* routinely screening with mammography (weak recommendation; moderate-quality evidence) 50: routinely recommend (weak recommendation; moderate-quality evidence)		50–69: every 2–3 years (weak recommendation; moderate-quality evidence) 70–74: Every 2–3 years (weak recommendation; low-quality evidence)	Recommend *not* routinely performing clinical breast exam (weak recommendation; low-quality evidence)	Recommend *not* advising women to routinely practice BSE (weak recommendation; moderate-quality evidence)

- Having "extremely" or "heterogeneously" dense breasts on mammograms
- Lifetime breast cancer risk greater than 15–25% as calculated using risk assessment tools

- Risk estimation

  - For those without clinical data, such as biopsy or mammogram data, family history can help identify those at risk of having a BRCA gene mutation. Recommended risk assessment tools are https://www.uspreventiveservicestaskforce.org/Page/Document/RecommendationStatementFinal/brca-related-cancer-risk-assessment-genetic-counseling-and-genetic-testing and include:

    - Referral Screening Tool (B-RST)
    - Ontario Risk Assessment Tool
    - Manchester Scoring System
    - Pedigree Assessment Tool
    - Family History Screen 7 (FHS-7)

  - For those with clinical data, such a biopsy or breast density data, the following tools may be helpful:

    - BCSC: https://tools.bcsc-scc.org/bc5yearrisk/calculator.htm
    - Tyrer-Cuzick: http://www.ems-trials.org/riskevaluator/

- Additional modes of breast cancer screening

  - Breast tomosynthesis (3D mammogram)

    - Takes many low-dose X-rays as it moves over the breast, which can be reconstructed into 3D images.
    - Sometimes uses more radiation than standard 2D mammography
    - Still requires breast compression
    - Preliminary data shows it may increase sensitivity and reduce false positives

- Not covered by all health insurance currently
- Both USPSTF and ACS currently report insufficient evidence to recommend for or against routine use of tomosynthesis for primary screening

- Breast ultrasound

  - Not routinely used for primary screening because of lower sensitivity in general population of average-risk women
  - Useful as adjuvant imaging in specific clinical settings: breast changes such as palpable lumps, dense breast tissue, and differentiation between fluid-filled cysts and solid masses

- MRI (magnetic resonance imaging)

  - Specific MRI machine required, with dedicated breast coils
  - Requires gadolinium contrast administration; some patients may have allergic reactions
  - Not routinely recommended for average-risk women because it misses some cancers identified with mammography and has high false-positive rate
  - May be routinely used to screen high-risk women (e.g., those with lifetime breast cancer risk of 20–25% based on risk factors, such as BRCA 1 or 2 mutation or history of high-dose chest radiation, or based on results of risk calculators such as the Tyrer-Cuzick http://www.ems-trials.org/riskevaluator), alternating with screening mammography

- Emerging technologies under investigation

  - Molecular breast imaging

    - Radioactive tracer injected into blood
    - Imaging then take up of the tracer in the breast is evaluated
    - Exposes whole body to radiation

- Still experimental technology
- Most likely utility is among women with a lump, abnormal mammogram, or dense breast tissue

  – Positive emission mammography

    - Radioactively tagged sugar is injected into the blood
    - Like a PET scan, a scanner examines uptake of the tracer in breast tissue
    - Exposes whole body to radiation
    - Clinical utility likely among women with breast cancer or breast lump

  – Electrical impedance imaging

    - Scans breast for electrical conductivity to identify abnormal cells
    - Performed by using small electrodes taped to breast
    - Does not use radiation or breast compression
    - Approved by FDA to help classify tumors identified on mammogram but still largely experimental

  – Elastography

    - Part of an ultrasound exam
    - Measures how firm/stiff breast tissue is compared with surrounding breast tissue
    - Requires mild compression
    - Still largely experimental

- Role of primary care providers

  - Can facilitate shared decision-making discussion given heterogeneity of guideline recommendations. Shared decision-making is defined as "an approach where clinicians and patients share the best available evidence when faced with the task of making decisions and where patients are supported to consider options, to achieve informed preferences." Resources to facilitate this discussion are:

- – USPSTF Clinical Summary of Mammography Screening Recommendations, Benefits and Harms: https://www.uspreventiveservicestask-force.org/Page/Document/ClinicalSummaryFinal/breast-cancer-screening1
- – Journal of the American Medical Association (JAMA) Patient Infographic Regarding Benefits and Harms of Screening: https://jamanetwork.com/journals/jama/fullarticle/2040228)
- – Canadian Task Force FAQs, Algorithm, and Risk/Benefit Summaries: https://canadiantaskforce.ca/tools-resources/breast-cancer-2/

- • Can identify women at high risk using risk calculators and refer for genetic counseling or intensive screening.
- • Serve as primary source of referrals to screening mammography

- – Additional resources

- • USPSTF: https://www.uspreventiveservicestaskforce.org/Page/Document/UpdateSummaryFinal/breast-cancer-screening1?ds=1&s=breast%20cancer
- • ACS:https://www.ncbi.nlm.nih.gov/pubmed/26501536
- • ACOG: https://www.acog.org/Clinical-Guidance-and-Publications/Practice-Bulletins/Committee-on-Practice-Bulletins-Gynecology/Breast-Cancer-Risk-Assessment-and-Screening-in-Average-Risk-Women
- • National Comprehensive Cancer Network (NCCN): https://www.nccn.org/professionals/physician_gls/pdf/breast-screening.pdf (available with free registration)
- • CTF: https://canadiantaskforce.ca/guidelines/pub-lished-guidelines/breast-cancer/

- *Cervical Cancer Screening*
  - Epidemiology
    - Approximately 12,800 new cases of cervical cancer diagnosed annually; prior to cervical cancer screening was one of the most common cancers in women
    - Approximately 4200 deaths annually from cervical cancer
    - As of 2014, approximately 256,000 women living with cervical cancer in the USA
  - Benefits and harms of screening
    - Benefits
      - Introduction of cervical cancer screening reduces rates of cervical cancer by 60–90% within 3 years of implementation in a screening naïve population
      - Cervical cancer mortality has decreased by 20–60% since the introduction of screening
    - Harms: may vary depending on type of screening, especially cytology vs. HPV testing. Though it is not clear whether overall harms increase or decrease when comparing cytology with HPV, below is a list of some harms associated with screening
      - Short-term psychological distress related to abnormal results
      - Surveillance procedures (i.e., colposcopy compared with biopsy) for minimally abnormal findings that result in increased rates of pain, bleeding, or discharge compared with minimally invasive surveillance
        - Pain: 39% vs. 15%, respectively
        - Bleeding: 47% vs. 17%, respectively
        - Discharge: 34% vs. 9%, respectively
      - Treatment procedures (i.e., cervical conization or loop electrosurgical procedures) for high-grade precancerous lesions that result in high rates of short- and long-term risks

- Pain: 67%
- Bleeding 87%
- Discharge: 63%
- Possible increase in perinatal mortality, preterm delivery prior to 34 weeks' gestation, and low birthweight

- Guidelines by organization (Table 3.3)

  - Overview

    - Papanicolaou screening remains the primary standard for screening, though multiple organizations are currently considering use of high-risk HPV testing (without cytology) as a possible method for primary screening
    - Current evidence does not indicate a clinically significant difference between conventional cytology and liquid cytology; as a result, they can be considered interchangeably in the screening recommendations
    - HPV testing methods vary; however, there do not appear to be clinically significant differences between different methods of high-risk testing (Table 3.3)

- Special populations

  - High risk that may require screening more often:

    - Diethylstilbestrol (DES) exposure in utero
    - Immunosuppressed women (organ transplant, HIV positive, long-term steroid use)
    - Precancers such as CIN2 or CIN3 in the past 20 years require screening to complete 20 years of surveillance

  - Low risk

    - Women who had hysterectomy with removal of uterus and cervix for indications other than cervical precancer or cervical cancer do not require further screening

TABLE 3.3 Cervical cancer screening guidelines (current as of May 2018)

Organization	Age to start screening	Age to end screening	Papanicolaou testing	HPV testing
USPSTF	21 years: (Grade A)	65 years: recommends against screening after age 65 if adequate screening *and* no high-risk conditions (Grade D)	21–65 years: every 3 years, without HPV co-testing (Grade A) 30–65 years: every 5 years with HPV co-testing (Grade A)	<30 years: recommends against primary HPV testing (Grade D) 30 years and older: consider HPV testing with cytology (draft revisions presented in 2017)
ACS	21 years:	65 years: no further screening recommended if adequate history of screening *and* no high-risk conditions	21–65 years: every 3 years if no HPV co-testing 30–65 years: preferred screening every 5 years with HPV co-testing	<30 years: does not recommend primary HPV testing 30–65 years: preferred screening is HPV co-testing with cytology
ACOG	Same as USPSTF			
AAFP or ACP	Same as USPSTF			
NCCN	Endorses ACS guidelines			

(continued)

TABLE 3.3 (continued)

Organization	Age to start screening	Age to end screening	Papanicolaou testing	HPV testing
Canadian Task Force on Preventive Health	<20 years: recommend *not* routine screening (strong recommendation; high-quality evidence) 20–24 years: recommend not routinely screening (weak recommendation; moderate-quality evidence) 25–29 years: recommend routine screening (weak recommendation; moderate-quality evidence) 30–69 years: recommend routine screening (strong recommendation; high-quality evidence)	≥70 years: cease routine screening if adequate screening (weak recommendation; low-quality evidence)	25–29: every 3 years (weak recommendation; moderate-quality evidence) 30–69: every 3 years (strong recommendation; high-quality evidence)	No recommendation for routine HPV testing (due for updated report in 2018)

- Women with prior HPV vaccination, though, should continue routine screening

- Inadequate screening

  - Women who have not had regular screening in 10 years prior to age 65 should have a screening test done. If negative, can stop

- Role of primary care providers

  - Perform Pap testing with or without HPV co-testing
  - Refer to gynecology or gynecology oncology for further evaluation of abnormal screening

- Additional resources

  - USPSTF: https://www.uspreventiveservicestaskforce.org/Page/Document/Recommendation StatementFinal/cervical-cancer-screening# consider
  - ACS: https://www.cancer.org/cancer/cervical-cancer/prevention-and-early-detection/cervical-cancer-screening-guidelines.html
  - CTF: https://canadiantaskforce.ca/guidelines/published-guidelines/cervical-cancer/

- *Colorectal Cancer (CRC) Screening*

  - Epidemiology:

    - Estimated 135,000 people diagnosed with colorectal cancer annually in the USA
    - Estimated over 50,000 deaths annually
    - As of 2014, estimated 1.3 million people in the USA living with colorectal cancer

  - Benefits and harms of screening for each method of screening (Table 3.4)
  - Screening guidelines for average-risk population (Table 3.5)
  - Decision aids may be useful to discuss benefits and harms of different strategies:

TABLE 3.4 Benefits and harms of colorectal cancer screening

Type of screening method	Benefits of screening	Harms of screening
Colonoscopy	Detection and removal of polyps Visualizes whole colon	Minor or major bleeding Dehydration or electrolyte imbalance with bowel prep Anesthesia risk Intestinal perforation
CT colonography	Less invasive No need for sedation	Accuracy depends on experience of radiologist Can miss small or flat polyps Incidental extracolonic findings
Sigmoidoscopy	Lower risk for harms with colonoscopy Requires minimal anesthesia	Visualizes only left colon Minor or major bleeding Intestinal perforation
Double-contrast barium enema		Less sensitive
Guaiac-based fecal occult blood test	Home-based Not invasive Inexpensive	Requires diet restrictions and multiple samples Lower sensitivity and specificity compared to FIT
Fecal immunohistochemical test (FIT)	Home-based Not invasive Inexpensive	False positives
Stool DNA	Increased sensitivity compared to FIT	Higher false-positive rates compared to FIT

TABLE 3.5 Colorectal cancer screening guidelines for average-risk individuals (current as of May 2018)

	USPSTF (AAFP follows)	ACP	ACS	AGA	Canadian Task Force
Age range (years)	50–75: grade A 75–85: grade C	50–75	Starting at 45 No specified age to end screening	Starting at 50 No specified age to end screening	50–74: strong 75+: weak
Recommended screening intervals by type of test					
Direct visualization					
Colonoscopy	10 years	10 years	10 years	10 years	NR for primary screening
CT colonography	5 years	NR	5 years	5 years	NR
Sigmoidoscopy	5 years 10 years if paired with FIT yearly	5 years	5 years	5 years	10 years
Double-contrast barium enema	NR	NR	5 years	NR	NR

(continued)

TABLE 3.5 (continued)

	USPSTF (AAFP follows)	ACP	ACS	AGA	Canadian Task Force
Stool-based					
Guaiac-based fecal occult blood test	Yearly	Yearly 3 years if paired with flex sig	Yearly	NR	2 years
Fecal immunohistochemical test (FIT)	Yearly	Yearly 3 years if paired with flex sig	Yearly	Yearly	2 years
Stool DNA	1–3 years		3 years	Interval undetermined	NR

NR not recommended

- For providers
  - CRICO: https://www.rmf.harvard.edu/Clinician-Resources/Guidelines-Algorithms/2014/CRC-Decision-Support-Tool
- For patients
  - http://www.colorectalcancerscreening4u.com/
  - AAFP: http://www.aafp.org/afp/2015/0115/p93-s1.html
  - CTF: https://canadiantaskforce.ca/wp-content/uploads/2016/05/ctfphccolorectal-cancerpatient-faqfinal-updated160222.pdf

- Special populations who are at higher risk for CRC often require more frequent screening intervals, earlier start age for screening, and are generally screened with direct visualization (e.g., colonoscopy). High-risk populations include:

  - Previous CRC or adenomatous polyps (e.g., tubular or villous)
  - Inflammatory bowel disease (e.g., ulcerative colitis or Crohn's disease)
  - History of CRC in one or more first-degree relatives (first-degree relative with CRC diagnosed before 60 or >2 first-degree relatives diagnosed at any age)
  - Hereditary syndromes predisposing to CRC (e.g., familial adenomatous polyposis or Lynch syndrome)

- Screening guidelines for populations at increased and high risk for CRC (Table 3.6):

  - Other populations: there is discussion regarding possible earlier CRC screening for black men and women, but this is controversial, and insurance coverage of screening prior to age 50 is variable. Decisions to start earlier screening should be considered after engaging patients in shared decision-making

TABLE 3.6 Colorectal cancer screening guidelines for high-risk individuals

	Age to start screening	Screening interval
Adenomatous polyp	Not applicable	Every 3–5 years depending on number and size of polyps
Inflammatory bowel disease	8 years after onset of pancolitis	Every 1–2 years
Family history of CRC	10 years prior to age of diagnosis of youngest case	Every 5 years
Personal history of CRC	Not applicable	Within 1 year of colon resection
Hereditary syndromes FAP Lynch syndrome	10–12 20–25	Yearly sigmoidoscopy Every 1–2 years

- Role of primary care providers:
  - Refer to specialist to perform direct visualization screening procedures (e.g., colonoscopy, CT colonography, etc.), or order/recommend stool-based screening tests (e.g., gFOBT, FIT, stool DNA)
  - Monitor screening intervals, depending on individual risk factors and type of test ordered
  - Refer to genetic counseling for high-risk individuals
- Additional resources:
  - USPSTF: https://www.uspreventiveservicestaskforce.org/Page/Document/RecommendationStatementFinal/colorectal-cancer-screening2
  - ACP: http://annals.org/aim/fullarticle/1090701/screening-colorectal-cancer-guidance-statement-from-american-college-physicians

- ACS: https://www.cancer.org/cancer/colon-rectal-cancer/detection-diagnosis-staging/acs-recommen-dations.html
- AGA: http://www.gastrojournal.org/article/S0016-5085(17)35599-3/fulltext
- AAFP: http://www.aafp.org/afp/2015/0115/p93.html
- CTF: https://canadiantaskforce.ca/guidelines/pub-lished-guidelines/colorectal-cancer/

- *Prostate Cancer Screening*
  - Epidemiology
    - Estimated over 161,000 men diagnosed with prostate cancer annually in the USA
    - Estimated 26,700 deaths annually
    - As of 2014, estimated 3.1 million men in the USA living with prostate cancer
  - Benefits and harms of screening for each type of screening
    - Prostate-specific antigen (PSA):
      - Benefits: may have potential mortality benefit
      - Harms: high positive rates lead to overdiagnosis and overtreatment, high false-negative rates, and anxiety. Treatment also often associated with sex-ual, urinary, or rectal complications
      - Landmark papers about PSA screening:
        - Prostate, Lung, Colorectal, and Ovarian (PLCO) Cancer Screening Trial. Conducted in the USA, the study found no differences in rate of deaths from prostate cancer between the control group with no PSA testing and the screening group who was offered annual PSA testing (for 6 years) and annual digital rectal exam (for 4 years). One limitation of the study was that over 50% of control group participants had a PSA by their 6th year of participation
        - European Randomized Study of Screening for Prostate Cancer. This European study found

20% reduction in mortality rates from prostate cancer among those in a screening group that were offered PSA screening about every 4 years compared with a control group who was not offered screening. They found that for every 1 prostate cancer death avoided, 48 additional men would undergo prostate cancer treatment. One limitation of this study is the heterogeneity of screening intervals used

- Digital rectal exam (DRE):
    - Benefits: unclear there are any benefits
    - Harms: physical discomfort; possible rectal bleeding

- Guidelines by organization

    - USPSTF: recommends against screening with PSA
    - AAFP: recommends against screening with PSA
    - ACP: recommends shared decision-making for men aged 55–69 years and recommends against PSA unless patients express clear preference for screening
    - ACS: recommends both PSA (every 2 years if PSA <2.5 ng/ml and yearly if PSA >2.5 ng/ml) and DRE; recommends shared decision-making for men ≥50 years who are at average risk
    - AUA: recommends shared decision-making for men aged 55–69 years who are at average risk and considers that PSA screening can be done every other year

- Decision aids for patients

    - ACP: http://annals.org/aim/fullarticle/1676184/ screening-prostate-cancer-guidance-statement-from-clinical-guidelines-committee-american
    - ACS: https://www.cancer.org/content/dam/cancer-org/cancer-control/en/booklets-flyers/testing-for-prostate-cancer.pdf

- Prostate Cancer Research Foundation (Europe): http://www.prostatecancer-riskcalculator.com/

- Special populations

  - Black men: ACS recommends to start shared decision-making about PSA screening for black men >45 years.
  - Those with family history of prostate cancer:

    - One first-degree relative diagnosed with prostate cancer before age 65, ACS recommends to start shared decision-making about PSA screening for men >45 years
    - >1 first-degree relative diagnosed with prostate cancer before age 65, ACS recommends to start shared decision-making about PSA screening for men >40 years

- Role of primary care providers

  - Shared decision-making discussions with patients about risks/benefits of screening with PSA
  - Identify patients who are at higher risk for prostate cancer

- Additional resources

  - USPSTF: https://www.uspreventiveservicestaskforce. org/Page/Document/RecommendationStatementFinal/ prostate-cancer-screening
  - AAFP: https://www.aafp.org/afp/2015/1015/p683. html
  - ACP: http://annals.org/aim/fullarticle/1676183/ screening-prostate-cancer-guidance-statement-from-clinical-guidelines-committee-american
  - ACS: https://www.cancer.org/cancer/prostate-cancer/ early-detection/acs-recommendations.html
  - AUA: http://www.auanet.org/guidelines/early-detection-of-prostate-cancer-(2013-reviewed-and-validity-confirmed-2015)

- *Lung Cancer Screening*
  - Epidemiology
    - Second most common cancer: over 222,000 people diagnosed with lung cancer annually in the USA
    - Leading cause of cancer deaths in the USA: estimated almost 156,000 deaths annually
    - As of 2014, an estimated 527,228 people in the USA are living with lung cancer
  - Benefits and harms of screening with low-dose computed tomography (LDCT)
    - Benefits
      - Twenty percent risk reduction in lung cancer mortality seen in National Lung Screening Trial (NLST)
    - Harms
      - High false-positive rates and subsequent downstream consequences due to further testing needed to confirm or disprove initial finding
      - Overdiagnosis
      - Incidental findings
      - Radiation exposure
  - Guidelines by organization
    - USPSTF: annual LDCT for patients 55–80 years old with >30 pack-year smoking history *and* who are current smokers or quit <15 years ago
    - AAPF: insufficient evidence to recommend for or against LDCT in persons at high risk based on age and smoking history
    - ACP: follows USPSTF guidelines
    - ACS: shared decision-making about lung cancer screening for patients 55–74 years old with >30 pack-year smoking history *and* who are current smokers or quit <15 years ago *and* who are in relatively good health

- ACCP (American College of Chest Physicians) and ATS (American Thoracic Society): LDCT in patients 55–74 years old with >30 pack-year smoking history *and* who are current smokers or quit <15 years ago *and* without severe comorbidity that would limit life expectancy
- CTF: annual LDCT up to three times for patients 55–74 years with ≥30 pack-year smoking history *and* who are current smokers or quit <15 years ago

– Guidance on decision-making

- USPSTF: patient information sheet (downloadable from webpage)
- ACS: patient information sheet http://onlinelibrary. wiley.com/store/10.3322/caac.21177/asset/21177_ftp. pdf?v=1&t=j9xmd6x6&s=77ac41edc4747405f2cf9bd e971697279a60b89f
- AHRQ: decision aid for patients and for healthcare professionals to use in shared decision-making with patients and information sheet for PCPshttps:// effectivehealthcare.ahrq.gov/decision-aids/ lung-cancer-screening/
- ATS: patient information booklet https://www.thoracic.org/patients/patient- resources/resources/decision-aid-lcs.pdf
- CTF: patient information and FAQ https://canadiantaskforce.ca/tools-resources/lung- cancer-2/lung-cancer-for-patients/

– Role of primary care providers

- Counsel smoking cessation for current smokers
- Engage in shared decision-making about LDCT screening for high-risk population
- Refer for yearly screening for high-risk patients who are interested in undergoing screening

- Additional resources

  - USPSTF: https://www.uspreventiveservicestaskforce. org/Page/Document/RecommendationStatementFinal/ lung-cancer-screening
  - AAFP: https://www.aafp.org/afp/2014/0715/od1.html
  - ACS: http://onlinelibrary.wiley.com/doi/10.3322/ caac.21172/full
  - ATS: https://www.thoracic.org/statements/resources/ lcod/implem-ldct-screening.pdf
  - CTF: https://canadiantaskforce.ca/guidelines/pub- lished-guidelines/lung-cancer/

- *Other Cancers*

  - Liver cancer

    - No recommendation for screening in the general population
    - High-risk individuals (i.e., those with cirrhosis from any cause, those with chronic Hep B infection regardless of cirrhosis) should consider screening for hepatocellular carcinoma (HCC) with blood testing (AFP) and liver ultrasound every 6–12 months

  - Melanoma

    - May consider regular total body skin examinations in individuals at high risk (i.e., dysplastic nevus syn- drome, strong family history of melanoma, personal history of melanoma)
    - Additional methods of screening high-risk individu- als include dermatoscopy (to evaluate areas of con- cern more thoroughly) or tracking of moles using mole mapping or total body photography

  - Ovarian

    - No major organizations (USPSTF, ACS, ACOG, NCCN) endorse routine screening in average-risk women

- May consider screening with transvaginal ultrasound and/or CA-125 blood test in women at high risk of developing ovarian cancer (i.e., BRCA gene mutation carriers and those with significant family history of ovarian cancer), though no reliable evidence that screening reduces mortality even in high-risk women

- Testicular
  - Screening is no longer recommended for males of any age
- Thyroid cancer
  - USPSTF recommends against routine screening of thyroid cancer and no longer recommends routine palpation of the thyroid gland during a physical examination
  - Consider screening in individuals at high risk of thyroid cancer, including those with family history of medullary thyroid cancer (MTC) with or without type 2 multiple endocrine neoplasia (MEN-2), with thyroid ultrasound, genetic testing for mutations increasing risk of MTC, or blood tests such as TSH, T3, T4, thyroglobulin, calcitonin, or CEA

References

Andriole GL, Crawford ED, Grubb RL 3rd, Buys SS, Chia D, Church TR, et al. Mortality results from a randomized prostate-cancer screening trial. New Engl J Med. 2009;360(13):1310–9.

Ashton-Prolla P, Giacomazzi J, Schmidt AV, Roth FL, Palmero EI, Kalakun L, et al. Development and validation of a simple questionnaire for the identification of hereditary breast cancer in primary care. BMC Cancer. 2009;9:283.

Canadian Task Force on Preventive Health Care. Grades of Recommendation, Assessment, Development, and Evaluation (GRADE) Working Group. 2011. http://www.canadiantask-force.ca/

Clinical practice guidelines we can trust. Graham R, Mancher M, Miller Wolman D, Greenfield S, Steinberg E, Editors. Washington, DC: The National Academies Press. 2011.

Elwyn G, Coulter A, Laitner S, Walker E, Watson P, Thomson R. Implementing shared decision making in the NHS. BMJ. 2010;341:c5146.

Evans DG, Eccles DM, Rahman N, Young K, Bulman M, Amir E, et al. A new scoring system for the chances of identifying a BRCA1/2 mutation outperforms existing models including BRCAPRO. J Med Genet. 2004;41(6):474–80.

Gilpin CA, Carson N, Hunter AG. A preliminary validation of a family history assessment form to select women at risk for breast or ovarian cancer for referral to a genetics center. Clin Genet. 2000;58(4):299–308.

Hoskins KF, Zwaagstra A, Ranz M. Validation of a tool for identifying women at high risk for hereditary breast cancer in population-based screening. Cancer. 2006;107(8):1769–76.

Jin J. Breast cancer screening: benefits and harms. JAMA. 2014;312(23):2585.

Myers ER, Moorman P, Gierisch JM, Havrilesky LJ, Grimm LJ, Ghate S, et al. Benefits and harms of breast cancer screening: a systematic review. JAMA. 2015;314(15):1615–34.

National Cancer Institute Surveillance Epidemiology, and End Results Program. Cancer stat facts: female breast cancer. https://seer.cancer.gov/statfacts/html/breast.html

Pace LE, Keating NL. A systematic assessment of benefits and risks to guide breast cancer screening decisions. JAMA. 2014;311(13):1327–35.

Revisiting Wilson and Jungner in the genomic age: a review of screening criteria over the past 40 years. World Health Organization. 2011.

Rex DK, Boland CR, Dominitz JA, Giardiello FM, Johnson DA, Kaltenbach T, et al. Colorectal cancer screening: recommendations for physicians and patients from the U.S. Multi-Society Task Force on Colorectal Cancer. Am J Gastroenterol. 2017;112(7):1016–30.

Schroder FH, Hugosson J, Roobol MJ, Tammela TL, Ciatto S, Nelen V, et al. Screening and prostate-cancer mortality in a randomized European study. New Engl J Med. 2009;360(13):1320–8.

Smith RA, Andrews KS, Brooks D, Fedewa SA, Manassaram-Baptiste D, Saslow D, et al. Cancer screening in the United States, 2017: a review of current American Cancer Society guidelines and current issues in cancer screening. CA Cancer J Clin. 2017;67(2):100–21.

Tyrer J, Duffy SW, Cuzick J. A breast cancer prediction model incorporating familial and personal risk factors. Stat Med. 2004;23(7):1111–30.

U.S. Preventive Service Task Force. Clinical Summary Breast Cancer: Screening. 2016. https://www.uspreventiveser-vicestaskforce.org/Page/Document/UpdateSummaryFinal/breast-cancer-screening1

Vachon CM, Pankratz VS, Scott CG, Haeberle L, Ziv E, Jensen MR, et al. The contributions of breast density and common genetic variation to breast cancer risk. J Natl Cancer Inst. 2015;107(5).

Wolf AM, Fontham ET, Church TR, Flowers CR, Guerra CE, LaMonte SJ, et al. Colorectal cancer screening for average-risk adults: 2018 guideline update from the American Cancer Society. CA Cancer J Clin. 2018;68:250–81.

Chapter 4
Cancer Diagnosis

Kimberly S. Peairs

Overview

Timeliness of a cancer diagnosis has been associated with better clinical and patient-reported outcomes. Primary care providers are often faced with a myriad of patient symptoms with the challenging expectation they will be able to discern those that require further evaluation with the appropriate diagnostic tests and referrals. While screening and surveillance efforts are aimed at identifying cancer when patients are asymptomatic, the majority of malignancies manifest with symptoms. This chapter will focus on the symptomatic presentations of malignancies and the diagnostic options for assessment.

Definitions of Key Cancer Diagnosis Terms

- *Cancer screening:* testing asymptomatic individuals to identify cancer at early stage

K. S. Peairs (✉)

Division of General Internal Medicine, Johns Hopkins University School of Medicine, Baltimore, MD, USA

e-mail: kpeairs@jhmi.edu

© Springer Nature Switzerland AG 2019   69

L. Nekhlyudov et al. (eds.), *Caring for Patients Across the Cancer Care Continuum*,

https://doi.org/10.1007/978-3-030-01896-2_4

- *Cancer surveillance:* close, timely monitoring for cancer in individuals who are at increased risk of disease (prior cancer, high risk)
- *Alarm symptoms:* more concerning for malignancy than other nonspecific symptoms. Still may be benign but warrant more timely evaluation. These may not be the presenting symptom for each cancer type but, if present, raise concern for cancer
- *Positive predictive value (PPV) of symptom:* the chance the patient has the cancer associated with the symptom when presenting to the primary care provider

  - PPV ≥ 5% may be highly predictive of underlying cancer (Box 4.1)
  - Age, gender, and comorbidities affect the PPV of symptoms (e.g., patients >65 are at higher risk for common tumors such as breast, prostate, and colorectal)

Box 4.1 Symptoms, Signs, or Tests with Positive Predictive Value >5% for Cancer

- Colorectal cancer – rectal bleeding, change in bowel habits, and iron deficiency anemia
- Urologic cancer – hematuria
- Prostate cancer – abnormal prostate examination
- Lung cancer – hemoptysis
- Esophageal cancer – dysphagia
- Breast cancer – breast lump
- Gynecologic malignancy – postmenopausal bleeding

Adapted from Shapley et al. (2010).

Epidemiology

- More than 1.6 million new cancer cases diagnosed in the USA yearly
- Overall cancer incidence rate is 20% higher for men than women

- The most common new cancer sites for women in the USA are:

    - Breast: 250,000/year (30%)
    - Lung: 105,000/year (12%)
    - Colorectal: 64,000/year (8%)
    - Uterine: 61,000/year (7%)
    - Thyroid: 42,000/year (5%)

- The most common new cancer sites for men in the USA are:

    - Prostate: 161,000/year (19%)
    - Lung: 116,000/year (14%)
    - Colorectal: 71,000/year (9%)
    - Urinary bladder: 60,000/year (7%)
    - Melanoma: 52,000/year (6%)

Assessment of Potential Cancer

There are important components for a timely diagnosis of cancer that include:

- Clarification of presenting symptoms and identification of alarm symptoms
- Recognizing risk factors of individual patients:

    - Age and gender
    - Prior malignancy
    - Prior radiotherapy or chemotherapy
    - Predisposing inflammatory disorders (e.g., ulcerative colitis, hepatitis C)
    - Environmental risk factors (e.g., HPV exposure, tobacco, asbestos, etc.)
    - Family history of cancer or known genetic predisposition

- Choosing appropriate test and/or referral to specialist for diagnostic evaluation

Specific Common Cancers

Breast Cancer

Risk Factors *Older age (>65)*, family history, early menarche, late menopause, nulliparity, prior biopsies (even benign), dense breasts on mammography, prior radiation, inherited genetic mutations, tobacco, excessive alcohol, and postmenopausal obesity.

Signs/Symptoms
- *Breast mass* is the most common reported symptom associated with cancer and should always be evaluated. Higher incidence of cancer in those >45
- Nipple changes (inversion or unilateral bloody discharge)
- Skin changes (redness, swelling, warmth) that persist may be seen with inflammatory cancer
- Change in size of the breast
- Breast pain is a common chief complaint in primary care but rarely related to breast cancer in absence of breast or axillary mass (more concerning if noncyclical)

Evaluation Options
- Palpable breast mass:-imaging evaluation is necessary to further characterize mass.

    - Diagnostic mammography (DM) for women ≥40 years. If negative or correlated image of mass is suspicious then targeted ultrasound may be used
    - Digital breast tomosynthesis (DBT or "3D" mammography) may increase sensitivity of testing and may be particularly helpful in women <40 years (may also be used in women >40 years). This is a modification of digital mammography and provides a three-dimensional image of the breast. Patient recall rates (callback for additional imaging) slightly reduced compared to DM (less false positive readings); however, increased num-

ber of biopsies may occur related to increased sensitivity
- Ultrasound is suggested as first imaging technique for assessment of palpable lump in women <30 years or if pregnant or lactating. If abnormal, then DM or DBT is indicated
- Any highly suspicious breast mass on imaging (e.g., spiculated soft tissue mass, grouped microcalcifications) should have core biopsy
- Any suspicious breast mass palpated should be biopsied, even if not visualized on imaging (refer to surgeon). Mammography should be done first to evaluate for other potential breast abnormalities
- Breast MRI is not first-line evaluation technique for breast mass. MRI may be useful for further clarification of inconclusive mammogram and no ultrasound-correlated abnormality

- Noncyclical, unilateral, or focal breast pain

  - Ultrasound for women <30 years, pregnant, or lactating
  - DM or DBT may be used for concerning ultrasound or women >30 years
  - Breast MRI is not first-line evaluation technique for breast mass. MRI may be useful for further clarification of inconclusive mammogram and no ultrasound-correlated abnormality

Prostate Cancer

Risk Factors Age >65, family history, inherited genetic mutations, race (African Americans are at higher risk)

Signs/Symptoms
- Lower urinary tract symptoms of nocturia, urinary frequency, hesitancy, or retention (similar to benign prostatic hypertrophy)

- Erectile dysfunction
- Hematuria
- Metastatic disease may present with weight loss and bone pain.

Evaluation Options
- Digital rectal exam (DRE) – evaluation for asymmetry or nodules
- Prostate-specific antigen (PSA) – if elevated, this may warrant further evaluation (particularly if associated with symptoms)

  - Confirmation of elevated PSA with repeat testing should occur before proceeding to biopsy as many will return to baseline within a month
  - In an average-risk man, a PSA $\geq$ 4 ng/ml should warrant biopsy

- PSA derivatives may be considered to help the specificity of screening:

  - Serum % free PSA – if PSA is between 4 and 10 ng/ml, a lower % free PSA is more suggestive of cancer
  - Prostate Health Index (PHI) >35 more suggestive of malignancy

- Referral for biopsy

  - Transrectal prostate biopsy should be done for any suspicious exam findings
  - Transrectal ultrasound (TRUS) guided biopsy may be used to further evaluate findings from DRE
  - Magnetic resonance imaging (MRI)-targeted prostate biopsy is being evaluated to improve accuracy; for patients who may be involved in active surveillance or patients with rising PSA and prior negative biopsy
  - If biopsy negative, close monitoring for rising PSA is necessary. This would be with repeat PSA and DRE at 6–12 months depending on risks and suspicion of malignancy

– Urine prostate cancer antigen 3 (PCa3) RNA test may be useful additional test for patients with negative prostate biopsy but persistently elevated PSA ≥4 ng/ml. If elevated, may suggest need for rebiopsy

Colorectal Cancer

Risk Factors Age > 50, male sex, family history, inherited genetic mutations, inflammatory bowel disease, adenomatous polyps, diabetes mellitus, obesity, tobacco, excessive alcohol, and increased intake of red or processed meats

Signs/Symptoms
- *Rectal bleeding* – high predictive value in patients ≥50 years old
- Change in bowel habits (constipation or diarrhea; change in caliber of stool)
- Weight loss or abdominal pain (lower predictive values)
- Increased likelihood of cancer if combination of symptoms
- Other concerning signs: abdominal mass and unexplained iron deficiency

Evaluation Options
- Referral for colonoscopy
- If incomplete colonoscopy, then may consider CT colonography (will need colonic prep and insufflation)
- Video endoscopy capsule after incomplete colonoscopy for symptom evaluation (data less clear)
- Use of flexible sigmoidoscopy and barium enema (even if combined) has lower yield rates than colonoscopy or CT colonography
- Tumor markers (CEA, CA 19-9, etc.) are *not* for diagnostic purposes. They are valuable in assessment and follow-up of patients with known colorectal cancer
- Abdominal/pelvis CT with IV and oral contrast if concerned for mass (avoid oral contrast if concern for obstruction)

Lung Cancer

Risk Factors Tobacco use or exposure, radon, occupational exposures (asbestos, arsenic, coal tar, chromium), outdoor pollution, poor cooking ventilation, older age ($\geq$50 years old), and family history

Signs/Symptoms
- *Hemoptysis* is an alarm symptom for pulmonary malignancy, particularly in older men or those with other constitutional symptoms (weight loss, anorexia, dyspnea)
- Chronic cough, dyspnea, and chest pain are nonspecific but in conjunction with risk factors warrant evaluation. Persistent infection may be secondary to obstructing mass
- Extension of pulmonary tumor may cause compressive symptoms such as superior vena cava syndrome, bone pain, or hoarseness (recurrent laryngeal nerve paralysis)
- Paraneoplastic syndromes may be present such as:

  - Endocrine: SIADH production, Cushing syndrome, hypercalcemia
  - Neurologic: neuropathy, Lambert-Eaton syndrome
  - Collagen-vascular: dermatomyositis, polymyositis, vasculitis
  - Skin: acanthosis nigricans, pruritus, Sweet's syndrome
  - Skeletal: hypertrophic osteoarthropathy

Evaluation Options
- Chest radiograph for initial symptoms. Comparison with prior radiographs for changes. If new lesion, pleural effusion, pleural nodularity, lymphadenopathy, post-obstruction pneumonia, or segmental or lobar atelectasis is present, CT should be performed
- Chest CT with contrast for suspected lung cancer (and upper abdomen); non-contrast CT is used for screening and monitoring of nodules (Box 4.2)

- PET or PET/CT may identify occult disease better than CT and used for evaluation of potential metastatic disease. May also help to differentiate benign versus malignant solitary pulmonary nodule. Data on survival improvement unclear
- Tissue diagnosis is necessary and approach is dependent on site of lesion (bronchoscopy, CT-guided transthoracic biopsy, mediastinal biopsy, pleural fluid sampling)

Box 4.2 Solitary Pulmonary Nodule: Finding on CT Suggestive of Malignancy
- Size >15 mm
- Irregular or speculated borders
- Upper lobe location
- Thick-walled cavitation
- Ground glass lesion that has (or develops) solid component
- Enlarging nodule

Gynecologic Cancers

Ovarian Cancer

Risk Factors Older age and postmenopausal, inherited genetic mutations, family history, prolonged hormone replacement therapy, pelvic inflammatory disease, and asbestos exposure

Signs/Symptoms
(Many are nonspecific but present over prior 12 months):

- Abdominal/pelvic distention or "bloating" and abdominal/pelvic pain
- Increased urinary urgency or frequency for over 1 month
- Early satiety or loss of appetite
- Unexplained weight loss, fatigue, or change in bowel habits
- New irritable bowel symptoms in patient >50 years old

Evaluation Options
- Abdominal/pelvic examination
- Abdominal/pelvic ultrasound
- CT (with contrast) or MRI (particularly if abnormal exam)
- CA125 tumor marker; other tumor markers may be considered such as alpha-fetoprotein (AFP) in women <35 years; beta-human chorionic gonadotropin (beta-hCG), and inhibin
- Evaluation by a gynecologic oncologist for concerning findings
- Tissue biopsy is necessary

Endometrial Cancer

Risk Factors Older age, unopposed estrogen use, tamoxifen use, family history, and obesity (of all malignancies, endometrial is most strongly associated).

Signs/Symptoms
- Postmenopausal bleeding (unexplained vaginal bleeding >12 months after menopause) is present in up to 90% cases of uterine cancer and should prompt immediate evaluation/referral to gynecology
- Heavy or irregular bleeding in premenopausal patients (although more commonly this is benign)
- Vaginal discharge, abdominal pain, and hematuria
- Anemia, thrombocytosis, and elevated blood glucose

Evaluation Options
- Abdominal/pelvic examination
- Pelvic ultrasound; if thickened endometrial stripe, then gynecologic referral
- Tissue may be obtained by endometrial biopsy

Cervical Cancer

Risk Factors Human papillomavirus (HPV), Immuno-suppression (HIV, organ transplant recipients), and in utero DES exposure

Signs/Symptoms
• Intermenstrual, postcoital, or postmenopausal bleeding
• Persistent vaginal discharge, hematuria, and abdominal pain

Evaluation Options
• Cervical examination with infection screen
• If suspicious lesion visualized, refer to gynecologist
• Cervical cytology should be obtained
• Consider other source if abnormal bleeding (uterine, ovarian)

Brain, Head, or Neck Cancer

Brain Cancer

Risk Factors Older age, radiation exposure, family history, inherited genetic susceptibility (neurofibromatosis 1 and 2, tuberous sclerosis, von Hippel-Lindau, Li-Fraumeni), and immunodeficiency (higher risk for lymphoma)

Signs/Symptoms
• Headache may be present in approximately half of patients with brain tumors (from primary or metastatic process) but more commonly not related to cancer. See "red flags" of headaches (Box 4.3)
• New onset of neurologic symptoms (seizure, mental status change, cranial nerve deficits, motor or sensory changes in central CNS pattern)

Box 4.3 Headache "Red Flags" Concerning for Malignancy

- New-onset headache in patient >age 50
- Sudden-onset headache
- Worsening or change in headache pattern
- Headache triggered by cough, bending over, or Valsalva
- Presence of other focal neurological signs or symptoms
- New headache in immunocompromised patient or if prior cancer

Evaluation Options
- Complete neurological and head examination (evaluate for papilledema)
- MRI with contrast; if contraindicated then CT
- Stereotactic needle biopsy versus open craniotomy for tissue diagnosis if thought to be primary tumor
- If concern for leptomeningeal spread or metastatic disease, lumbar puncture for cytology

Head or Neck Cancer

Risk Factors Tobacco (smoked and smokeless), excessive alcohol use, older age, HPV infection, and radiation exposure

Signs/Symptoms

- Will vary based on anatomical location: pharynx, oral cavity, larynx, nasal cavity and paranasal sinuses, salivary glands, and thyroid

  - *Oral cavity tumors*: non-healing ulcers, dysphagia, odynophagia, pain referred to ear
  - *Pharyngeal tumors*: dysphagia, odynophagia, otalgia, hearing loss, neck mass

- *Laryngeal tumors*: hoarseness, cough, stridor, hemopty-sis, lymphadenopathy
- *Sinus tumors*: epistaxis, unilateral nasal obstruction, facial pain, protracted otitis media

- Rapidly enlarging neck mass may be a lymph node (firm, fixed are suspicious) or primary tumor

Evaluation Options
- Thorough examination of the head and neck with palpation and attention to thyroid examination
- Otolaryngology evaluation for direct flexible laryngoscopy with visualization of posterior pharynx and vocal cord mobility
- Contrast-enhanced CT imaging of the head or neck may be used for evaluation of other structures or extent of tumor involvement
- MRI may provide better soft tissue imaging and complement CT
- Referral to specialist for further evaluation
- PET/CT may be superior for initial staging once diagnosis is made
- Chest imaging may be warranted for high-risk patients (tobacco use) and hoarseness
- Fine-needle aspiration biopsy may be least invasive technique to obtain tissue diagnosis
- Thyroid masses should be evaluated with ultrasound, and fine-needle biopsy may be performed on suspicious nodules

Upper Gastrointestinal or Pancreatic Cancers

Risk Factors
Esophageal – tobacco and alcohol use, age > 55, male sex, Barrett's esophagus, chronic gastroesophageal reflux, esopha-

geal injury, HPV, and atrophic gastritis (seen with pernicious anemia).

Gastric – age > 50, male sex, *H. pylori* infection, atrophic gastritis, tobacco use, ethnic predisposition (Asian > Western countries), and inherited genetic disorders.

Signs/Symptoms
- *Dysphagia* (high PPV), odynophagia, early satiety or weight loss, and chest pain can be seen with esophageal malignancy
- Solid food dysphagia may precede liquid dysphagia
- Hoarseness later in disease if recurrent laryngeal nerve involved
- Chronic dyspepsia in conjunction with other "alarm features," such as unintentional weight loss, dysphagia, odynophagia, hematemesis, or in higher-risk patients (tobacco use, age > 45), should prompt evaluation for esophageal or gastric malignancy
- Dysphagia, epigastric pain, nausea, and weight loss are the most common symptoms for gastric cancer (but often not until advanced disease). Occult bleeding may also occur

Evaluation Options
- Referral to gastroenterologist for upper endoscopy
- Biopsy of abnormal areas; may consider biopsy mapping of non-targeted lesions for those at high risk

Pancreatic Cancer

Risk Factors Tobacco use, family history, inherited genetic predisposition, chronic pancreatitis, obesity, type II diabetes, occupational exposures, older age, male sex, and African American > Caucasian.

Signs/Symptoms
- Most are asymptomatic until advanced disease
- Abdominal pain, weight loss, and jaundice are the most common findings

- Head of pancreas tumors: jaundice with pruritus, pale-colored stools, and dark urine
- Body or tail of pancreas tumors: pain and weight loss
- Painless jaundice often presents secondary to resectable tumors
- "Atypical diabetes": –sudden onset of glucose intolerance in thin older adults may be an early sign
- Abdominal mass, ascites at later stages: left supraclavicular lymphadenopathy (Virchow's node) if metastatic spread

Evaluation Options
- Laboratory assessment to include liver function tests, bilirubin
- Abdominal imaging with pancreatic protocol CT (with contrast) preferred over abdominal ultrasound if suspicion is high
- Magnetic resonance cholangiopancreatography (MRCP) may be used for better visualization of biliary tree, liver, and vascular structures
- Endoscopic ultrasound (EUS) helpful for direct visualization and fine-needle aspiration (FNA) biopsy of area
- Endoscopic retrograde cholangiopancreatography (ERCP) is used less in era of EUS. Biopsy and brushings can be done at time of evaluation
- If unable to access with EUS, CT-guided biopsy may be considered

Tumor marker (CA 19-9) specificity is limited and sensitivity is related to tumor size. Not used as a diagnostic tool but helpful for follow-up.

Genitourinary Cancers

Bladder Cancer

Risk Factors Older age, male sex, Caucasian race, tobacco use, chemical exposures (dyes, diesel), arsenic, family history, inherited genetic predisposition, and radiation and chemotherapy (cyclophosphamide)

Signs/Symptoms
- Painless hematuria (more commonly gross bleeding)
- Frequency, urgency, and dysuria (but are nonspecific)
- Pain in pelvic region if advanced disease
- Unexplained microscopic hematuria (evaluate for infection first)

Evaluation Options
- If patient >40 years, unexplained hematuria work-up is indicated
- If no apparent source, the entire genitourinary tract should be assessed (renal, bladder, urethra)
- Urinalysis for hemoglobin, white cells, and red cells
- Cystoscopy for evaluation of bladder (may also obtain urine cytology with cystoscopy)
- Lower diagnostic yield from voided urine cytology compared to those obtained during cystoscopy

Renal Cancer

Risk Factors Tobacco use, obesity, male sex, family history, inherited genetic mutations, and chemical exposures (cadmium, herbicides, organic solvents)

Signs/Symptoms
- Usually asymptomatic until late presentation
- Hematuria (macroscopic), abdominal mass, and pain
- Weight loss, malaise, and anorexia may be early signs
- Anemia may precede diagnosis (consist with anemia of chronic disease)
- Men may develop new scrotal varicoceles; edema may come from IVC extension
- Paraneoplastic syndromes may be seen with metastatic disease (neurologic, cutaneous, rheumatologic, hepatic, metabolic)
- Laboratory abnormalities may include hypercalcemia, erythrocytosis, thrombocytosis, and amyloidosis

Evaluation Options
- Ultrasonography is less sensitive for renal mass but helpful to evaluate cyst vs. solid tumor
- CT with and without IV contrast
- MRI may be used if CT contrast contraindicated
- For solitary renal masses, partial or complete nephrectomy is suggested

Testicular Cancer

Risk Factors Undescended testicle, family history, HIV, and Caucasian race

Signs/Symptoms
- Enlarging testicular mass (often painless)
- "Scrotal heaviness"
- Ten percent may be caused by primary malignancies that are extragonadal: retroperitoneal (back pain or abdominal mass) and mediastinal (shortness of breath, chest pain, vena cava obstruction)

Evaluation Options
- History and physical examination of mass
- Ultrasound of testicular region
- Laboratory tests to include alpha-fetoprotein (AFP), beta-HCG, chemistry profile, and lactate dehydrogenase
- Referral to urologist

Lymphoma

Risk Factors *Hodgkin lymphoma*: early or late adulthood, family history, and immunocompromised state.

Non-Hodgkin lymphoma (NHL): older age, Caucasian, living in developed country, chemical exposures (chemotherapy, herbicides, benzenes), radiation exposure, certain viral or bacterial infections (chronic inflammation), and immunosuppression.

Signs/Symptoms
- Often nonspecific constitutional symptoms of fever, night sweats, weight loss, or fatigue
- Rare symptom is alcohol-induced pain (discomfort in areas of tumor after ingestion) in Hodgkin
- Asymptomatic neck mass with Hodgkin or lymphadenopathy elsewhere; concerning if lymphadenopathy >6 weeks, enlarging lymph nodes, lymph node >2 cm, or associated constitutional symptoms
- Extranodal disease in NHL may cause symptoms as first presentation (bone, liver, adrenals, brain)
- There is wide variation in NHL types with some indolent and others aggressive
- Splenomegaly should warrant further evaluation.

Evaluation Options
- Laboratory evaluation to include comprehensive metabolic panel, complete blood count with platelets, lactate dehydrogenase, erythrocyte sedimentation rate
- Contrast-enhanced CT of the chest, abdomen, and pelvis
- PET/CT (skull base to mid-thigh)
- Serum immunohistochemistry (flow cytometry)
- Excisional biopsy of lymph node recommended
- Core needle biopsy with immunohistochemistry as alternative

Skin Cancer

Risk Factors Excessive sun exposure during childhood, fair-skinned phenotype, presence of atypical nevi, family history of melanoma, and inherited genetic predisposition

Signs/Symptoms (for Melanoma)
- A – asymmetry
- B – border irregularity
- C – color variability

- D – diameter >6 mm
- E – evolving lesion (change in size, shape, and color, becomes tender and pruritic, or presence of bleeding)

Evaluation Options
- Referral for surgical resection (Table 4.1)

TABLE 4.1 Additional presenting signs or symptoms of malignancy

Presentation	Potential malignancy

Unintentional weight loss (more than 5% of body weight over 6–12 months)
    May be from biochemical or structural etiologies
    Often presents with abnormal exam or laboratory tests
	Gastrointestinal
	Hepatobiliary
	Hematologic
	Lung
	Breast
	Genitourinary
	Ovarian
	Prostate

Fever – recurring May also have night sweats	Hodgkin lymphoma Non-Hodgkin lymphoma Leukemia Renal cell Hepatic tumors (primary or metastatic)
Bone pain – bone marrow involvement or metastatic lesions Hypertrophic osteoarthropathy (digital clubbing, periosteal thickening on X-ray, joint effusion)	Multiple myeloma Lymphoma Sarcoma Leukemia Metastatic spread (common in the lung, breast, and prostate) Lung – hypertrophic osteoarthropathy

Bleeding
    Petechiae, ecchymoses
    Mucous membrane bleeding
	Leukemia

(continued)

TABLE 4.1 (continued)

Presentation	Potential malignancy
Deep vein thrombosis or pulmonary embolism (hypercoagulable disorder)	Ovarian Pancreatic Primary hepatic Brain Breast, colon, and lung also prevalent
Back pain – concerning if prior history of cancer, age ≥ 50, pain >1 month with conservative therapy, weight loss, and elevated inflammatory markers	Pancreatic may present with referred pain Multiple myeloma Hodgkin lymphoma Non-Hodgkin lymphoma Prostate Breast Lung
Soft tissue mass	Sarcoma

Disparities and Special Populations

• Influence of ethnicity/race on diagnosis of cancer:

  – African Americans have the highest mortality from major cancer sites (breast, lung, colorectal, prostate, stomach, cervical)
  – Potential reason for worse outcomes:

    • Variation in use or barriers to cancer screening
    • Different tumor biology
    • Patient's lack of awareness of symptoms
    • Barriers/delays in seeking care or receiving referrals

• High-risk groups

  – May have to consider more aggressive evaluation of symptom presentation
  – Inherited genetic predispositions (see Chap. 2)

    • Example: BRCA1 and BRCA2

  – Immunocompromised patients

  • Example: transplant patients on chronic immunosuppression and HIV

Cancer Diagnosis and Role of Primary Care

• The time from when a patient detects a potential cancer symptom and when they present for medical evaluation is variable. Access to and a relationship with a primary care provider may help expedite evaluation

• Adequate skills or knowledge for appropriate evaluation is necessary for timely diagnosis

• Some cancers present with symptoms that are present in benign conditions and nonspecific, making them a diagnostic challenge

• The primary care provider must identify "alarm symptoms" for expedited evaluation but be vigilant for more subtle symptom presentations that warrant further testing and referral to subspecialists

• Communication with the patient throughout the evaluation with clear follow-up plans ("safety netting"), particularly for non-diagnostic or equivocal tests (Fig. 4.1)

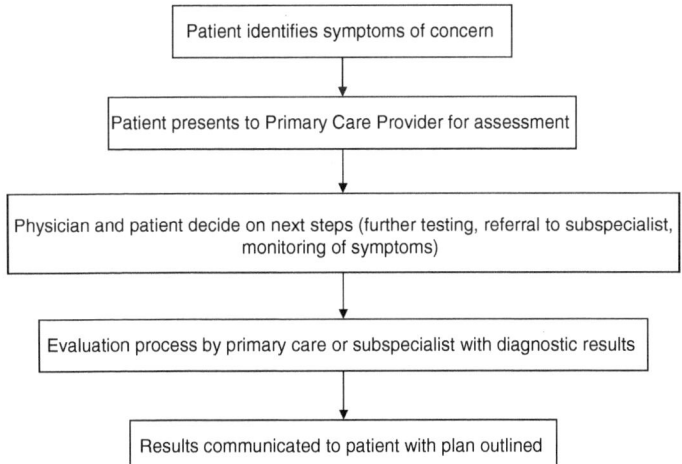

FIGURE 4.1 Role of primary care provider in cancer diagnosis

Additional Resources

- American Cancer Society. https://www.cancer.org/cancer/all-cancer-types.html. Accessed 16 May 2018.
- Johns Hopkins Medical Imaging Order Wisely Pocket Guide. https://www.hopkinsmedicine.org/imaging/_documents/order-wisely-pocket-guide.pdf. Accessed 16 May 2018.
- National Comprehensive Cancer Network Clinical Guidelines https://www.nccn.org/professionals/physician_gls/default.aspx#detection. Accessed 16 May 2018.
- NICE. Suspected cancer: recognition and referral. http://www.nice.org.uk/guidance/ng12. Accessed 16 May 2018.

References

American College of Radiology:https://acsearch.acr.org/docs/69482/Narrative/. Accessed 16 May 2018.

Expert Panel on Breast Imaging: Moy L, Heller SL, Bailey L, D'Orsi C, DiFlorio RM, Green ED, et al. ACR Appropriateness Criteria Palpable Breast Masses. J Am Coll Radiol. 2017;14(5S):S203–24.

Fojo AT. Cancer screening: still a work in progress. Semin Oncol. 2017: 44(1).

Hamilton W. The CAPER studies: five case-control studies aimed at identifying and quantifying the risk of cancer in symptomatic primary care patients. Br J Cancer 2009; 101: S80–S86.

Hamilton W, Walter F, Rubin G, Neal R. Improving early diagnosis of symptomatic cancer. Nat Rev Clin Oncol. December 2016;13:740–49.

Koo M, Hamilton W, Walter F, Rubin G, Lyratzopoulos G. Symptoms signatures and diagnostic timeliness in cancer patients: a review of current evidence. Neoplasia. 2018;20:165–74.

Martins T, Hamilton W. The influence of ethnicity on diagnosis of cancer. Fam Pract. 2016;33:325–6.

Nekhlyudov L, Latosinsky S. The interface of primary and oncology specialty care: from symptoms to diagnosis. J Natl Cancer Inst Monogr. 2010;40:11–7.

Peairs KS, Nekhlyudov L. Does my patient have cancer? Presenting symptoms. In: DeVita VT, Lawrence TS, Rosenberg SA, editors. Oncology in primary care. Philadelphia: Lippincott, Williams & Wilkins. 2013.

Seigel R, Miller K, Jemal A. Cancer Statistics, 2017. CA Cancer J Clin. 2017;67:7–30.

Shapley M, Mansell G, Jordan JL, Jordan KP. Positive predictive values of ≥ 5% in primary care for cancer: systematic review. Br J Gen Pract. 2010;60(578):e366–77.

Chapter 5
Cancer Treatment

Jenny J. Lin

Overview

Cancer treatment is evolving rapidly with many new options now available. This chapter reviews some of the basics of cancer treatment, including chemotherapy, hormonal therapy and immunotherapy, as well as common acute treatment toxicities and management suggestions. Primary care providers should have familiarity with these terms so that they have greater understanding of treatment plans, can help their patients in decision-making and clearly communicate with oncology colleagues.

Definitions

There are a number of terms that are commonly used during cancer treatment. Primary care providers should have familiarity with such terms so that they are able to have a greater understanding of the treatment plans, help their patients in

J. J. Lin (✉)
Division of General Internal Medicine,
Icahn School of Medicine at Mount Sinai, New York, NY, USA
e-mail: Jenny.Lin@mountsinai.org

© Springer Nature Switzerland AG 2019   93
L. Nekhlyudov et al. (eds.), *Caring for Patients Across the Cancer Care Continuum*,
https://doi.org/10.1007/978-3-030-01896-2_5

decision-making, and be able to communicate with their oncology colleagues. These terms are described below.

- *Performance status*: assesses functional status to determine which patients may benefit from treatment, Eastern Cooperative Oncology Group (ECOG) performance status often used, and patients with ECOG scores >2 less likely to benefit from chemotherapy:

  - ECOG 0: Fully active, able to carry on all pre-disease performance without restriction
  - ECOG 1: Restricted in physically strenuous activity but ambulatory and able to carry out work of a light or sedentary nature, e.g., light house work, office work
  - ECOG 2: Ambulatory and capable of all self-care but unable to carry out any work activities; up and about >50% of waking hours
  - ECOG 3: Capable of only limited self-care; confined to bed or chair >50% of waking hours
  - ECOG 4: Completely disabled; cannot carry on any self-care; totally confined to bed or chair

- *Staging:* describes the severity of a patient's cancer based on the size of the primary tumor and extent of spread (whether there is lymph node involvement or metastases). Staging allows the healthcare team to estimate prognosis and determine treatment plans and is often required for establishing eligibility in clinical trials.

  - Types of staging:

    - *Clinical*: extent of cancer determined based on physical examination, imaging tests, and biopsies of affected areas
    - *Pathologic*: determined after surgery that removes tumor or explores extent of cancer; combines results of both clinical staging (physical exam and imaging) with pathology results of surgical excision
    - *Post-therapy (post-neoadjuvant)*: extent of cancer remaining after patient has received treatment with systemic (chemotherapy or hormone therapy) and/or radiation therapy prior to surgery or where no sur-

gery was performed; assessed by either clinical and/ or pathologic staging

- *Restaging*: extent of disease cancer recurrence; helps determine treatment options after recurrence

- The TNM Staging System is based on:

  - Extent/size of the primary tumor (T): T0–T4
  - Extent of spread to the lymph nodes (N): N0–N3
  - Metastasis (M): M0 (absent) vs. M1 (present)

- General stages vary depending on tumor type/organ (see Table 5.1):

  - Stage 0: noninvasive cancer or carcinoma in situ
  - Stage I: localized primary tumor, tends to be completely resectable
  - Stage II: tumor still contained but larger than in stage I, may also have some lymph node involvement
  - Stage III: evidence of extension of primary tumor with local invasion or extension into deeper structures, with possible lymph node involvement
  - Stage IV: presence of distant metastases
  - Stage 0–II are generally considered localized, stage III is regional, and stage IV is distant

- Other factors affecting stage:

  - Cell type (e.g., squamous, ductal, glandular [adenocarcinoma], lobular, etc.)
  - Tumor grade: reflects degree of cell differentiation seen on pathological specimen, usually graded on a scale from 1 (low-grade) to 4 (high-grade)

    - Low-grade: well-differentiated tumors that are usually slower-growing and less likely to metastasize
    - Intermediate grade: moderately differentiated tumor
    - High-grade: poorly differentiated or undifferentiated tumors that are often more aggressive
    - Note: in prostate cancer, Gleason score refers to tumor grade and usually ranges from 6 (low-grade) to 10 (high-grade/aggressive)

TABLE 5.1 Survival and Incidence by Cancer Type

Cancer type	Incidence (per 100,000/yr) % of total	5-year survival rates
Breast	124.9	89.7%
Localized	62%	98.9%
Regional	31%	85.2%
Distant	6%	26.9%
Unstaged	2%	53.2%
Colorectal	40.1	64.9%
Localized	39%	89.9%
Regional	35%	71.3%
Distant	21%	13.9%
Unstaged	4%	35.4%
Genitourinary		
Bladder	19.8	77.3%
In situ	51%	95.7%
Localized	34%	70.1%
Regional	7%	35.2%
Distant	4%	5.0%
Unstaged	3%	45.7%
Prostate	119.8	98.6%
Localized	79%	100%
Regional	12%	100%
Distant	5%	29.8%
Unstaged	4%	81.2%
Renal	15.6	74.1%
Localized	65%	92.6%

TABLE 5.1 (continued)

Cancer type	Incidence (per 100,000/yr) % of total	5-year survival rates
Regional	16%	66.7%
Distant	16%	11.7%
Unstaged	3%	38.0%
Gynecologic		
Cervical	7.4	67.1%
Localized	56%	91.5%
Regional	36%	57.1%
Distant	14%	17.3%
Unstaged	4%	52.2%
Endometrial	25.7	81.3%
Localized	67%	95.3%
Regional	21%	68.5%
Distant	9%	16.2%
Unstaged	4%	50.3%
Ovarian	11.7	46.5%
Localized	15%	92.5%
Regional	20%	73.0%
Distant	60%	28.9%
Unstaged	6%	25.1%
Head and neck		
Oropharyngeal	11.2	64.5%
Localized	30%	83.7%
Regional	47%	64.2%

(continued)

TABLE 5.1 (continued)

Cancer type	Incidence (per 100,000/yr) % of total	5-year survival rates
Distant	19%	38.5%
Unstaged	4%	47.9%
Hematologic		
Leukemia	13.7	60.6%
Lymphoma (non-Hodgkin)	19.1	71.0%
Localized	28%	82.9%
Regional	15%	75.0%
Distant	50%	63.4%
Unstaged	8%	69.2%
Multiple myeloma	6.6	49.6%
Localized	5%	71.0%
Distant	95%	48.4%
Lung	55.8	18.1%
Localized	16%	55.6%
Regional	22%	28.9%
Distant	57%	4.5%
Unstaged	5%	7.5%
Thyroid	14.2	98.2%
Localized	68%	99.9%
Regional	27%	98.0%
Distant	4%	56.4%
Unstaged	2%	88.6%

- Tumor location
- Tumor markers (see Table 5.2):

    - Can include substances produced by tumors or by normal cells in response to tumors, in addition to patterns of gene expression or DNA rearrangement
    - Used to help with diagnosis, prognosis, and evaluation of treatment response/cancer progression

- *Treatment intent*

    - *Adjuvant*: treatment given after primary treatment to increase effectiveness of treatment and to decrease risk of cancer recurrence and/or prolong survival
    - *Curative*: treatment given to eradicate cancer cells
    - *Neoadjuvant*: treatment given prior to surgery with goal to shrink tumor prior to resection
    - *Palliative*: treatment given for symptom management and/or to control cancer progression but not to cure cancer; can prolong survival and/or improve quality of life

Treatment Types

- *Chemotherapy*: systemic treatment often delivered intravenously but some are given orally or intramuscular; often used in *adjuvant* or *neoadjuvant* setting, can also be used for *palliative treatment*. Major classes of chemotherapy include:
    - *Alkylating agents*: oldest class of chemotherapy, not cell-cycle specific, prevents cell division by causing cross-linkage of DNA strands, abnormal base pairing, or strand breaks, generally best for treating slow-growing cancers

        - Ethylenimines: hexamethylmelamine, thiotepa
        - Mustard gas derivatives: busulfan, chlorambucil, cyclophosphamide, ifosfamide, mechlorethamine, melphalan

TABLE 5.2 Tumor Markers

Tumor marker	Cancer type	Tissue	Purpose
ALK gene (rearrangement and overexpression)	Non-small cell lung cancer Anaplastic large cell lymphoma	Tumor	Treatment decision-making Prognosis
Alpha-fetoprotein (AFP)	Liver cancer Germ cell tumors	Blood	Liver cancer: diagnosis and response to treatment Germ cell tumors: stage, prognosis, and treatment response
Beta-2 microglobulin (B2M)	Multiple myeloma CLL Lymphomas	Blood Urine CSF	Prognosis Treatment response
Beta-hCG	Choriocarcinoma Germ cell tumors	Blood Urine	Stage Prognosis Treatment response
BRCA1 and *BRCA2* gene mutation	Breast cancer Ovarian cancer	Blood	Targeted therapy hard return Treatment decision-making
BCR-ABL fusion gene (Philadelphia chromosome)	CML ALL AML	Blood Bone marrow	Diagnosis confirmation Targeted therapy response prediction Disease status monitoring
BRAF V600 mutations	Melanoma (cutaneous) Colorectal cancer	Tumor	Targeted therapy treatment decision-making
C-kit/CD117	GIST Melanoma (mucosal)	Tumor	Diagnosis Treatment decision-making
CA15-3/CA 27-29	Breast cancer	Blood	Treatment response Disease recurrence

TABLE 5.2 (continued)

Tumor marker	Cancer type	Tissue	Purpose
CA19-9	Pancreatic cancer Gallbladder cancer Cholangiocarcinoma Gastric cancer	Blood	Treatment response
CA-125	Ovarian cancer	Blood	Diagnosis Treatment response Disease recurrence
Calcitonin	Medullary thyroid cancer	Blood	Diagnosis Treatment response Disease recurrence
Carcinoembryonic antigen (CEA)	Colorectal cancer	Blood	Treatment response Disease recurrence
CD20	Non-Hodgkin lymphoma	Blood	Targeted therapy treatment decision-making
Chromogranin A (CgA)	Neuroendocrine tumors	Blood	Diagnosis Treatment response Disease recurrence
Chromosomes 3, 7, 17 and 9p21	Bladder cancer	Urine	Disease recurrence
Circulating tumor cells of epithelial origin	Metastatic breast, prostate, and colorectal cancers	Blood	Prognosis Treatment decision-making
Cytokeratin fragment 21-1	Lung cancer	Blood	Disease recurrence
EGFR gene mutation	Non-small cell lung cancer	Tumor	Treatment decision-making Prognosis
Estrogen receptor (ER) and progesterone receptor (PR)	Breast cancer	Tumor	Treatment decision-making Targeted treatment

(continued)

TABLE 5.2 (continued)

Tumor marker	Cancer type	Tissue	Purpose
Fibrin/fibrinogen	Bladder cancer	Urine	Treatment response Disease progression
HE4	Ovarian cancer	Blood	Treatment decision-making Disease progression Disease recurrence
HER2/neu gene amplification or protein overexpression	Breast cancer Gastric cancer GE junction adenocarcinoma	Tumor	Targeted therapy treatment decision-making
Immunoglobulins	Multiple myeloma Waldenstrom macroglobulinemia	Blood Urine	Diagnosis Treatment response Disease recurrence
KRAS gene mutation	Colorectal cancer Non-small cell lung cancer	Tumor	Targeted therapy treatment decision-making
Lactate dehydrogenase (LDH)	Germ cell tumors Lymphoma Leukemia Melanoma Neuroblastoma	Blood	Stage Prognosis Treatment response
Neuron-specific enolase (NSE)	Small cell lung cancer Neuroblastoma	Blood	Diagnosis Treatment response
Nuclear matrix protein 22	Bladder cancer	Urine	Treatment response
Programmed death ligand 1 (PD-L1)	Non-small cell lung cancer	Tumor	Targeted therapy treatment decision-making
Prostate-specific antigen (PSA)	Prostate cancer	Blood	Diagnosis Treatment response Disease recurrence

TABLE 5.2 (continued)

Tumor marker	Cancer type	Tissue	Purpose
Thyroglobulin	Thyroid cancer	Blood	Treatment response Disease recurrence
Urokinase plasminogen activator (uPA) and plasminogen activator inhibitor (PAI-1)	Breast cancer	Tumor	Prognosis Treatment decision-making
5-Protein Signature (OVA1®)	Ovarian cancer	Blood	Diagnosis (for suspicious pelvic mass)
21-Gene signature (Oncotype DX®)	Breast cancer	Tumor	Recurrence risk
70-Gene signature (Mammaprint®)	Breast cancer	Tumor	Recurrence risk

- Nitrosoureas (can cross blood-brain barrier): carmustine, fotemustine, lomustine, semustine, streptozotocin
- Platinum based: carboplatin, cisplatin, oxaliplatin
- Tetrazines: altretamine, dacarbazine, procarbazine, mitozolomide, temozolomide

- *Antimetabolites*: have similar structure to folic acid or nucleotides and either block enzymes required for DNA synthesis or when incorporated into DNA induce damage and lead to apoptosis

  - Folic acid antagonist: methotrexate, pemetrexed
  - Purine antagonist: 6-mercaptopurine (6-MP), 6-thioguanine
  - Pyrimidine antagonist: 5-fluorouracil (5-FU), floxuridine, cytarabine, capecitabine (Xeloda), gemcitabine
  - Adenosine deaminase inhibitor: cladribine, fludarabine, nelarabine, pentostatin

- *Antitumor antibiotics*: many derived from *Streptomyces*, not cell-cycle specific, generally work by binding DNA and preventing RNA synthesis

  - Anthracyclines: aclarubicin, doxorubicin, daunorubicin, epirubicin, mitoxantrone, idarubicin, pirarubicin
  - Others: actinomycin, bleomycin, mitomycin

- *Plant alkaloids*: derived from plants, many are cell-cycle specific, blocking replication in the S or M phase

  - Topoisomerase inhibitors prevent normal unwinding of DNA during replication or transcription
    - Camptothecin analogs: irinotecan, topotecan
    - Podophyllotoxins: Etoposide, teniposide

  - Taxanes prevent microtubule disassembly: paclitaxel, docetaxel
  - Vinca alkaloids prevent microtubule formation: vincristine, vinblastine, vinorelbine, vindesine, vinflunine

- *Others*

  - Antimicrotubule: estramustine
  - Enzymes: asparaginase, pegaspargase
  - Retinoids: bexarotene, isotretinoin, tretinoin
  - Ribonucleotide reductase inhibitor: hydroxyurea
  - Steroid inhibitor: mitotane

- *Hormonal therapy:* also called endocrine therapy, often used as adjuvant therapy for hormone-sensitive tumors (most often breast and prostate)

  - *Androgen deprivation therapy (ADT)*: mostly used in prostate cancer

    - Antiandrogens: block testosterone; examples include bicalutamide, flutamide, and nilutamide
    - Gonadotropin-releasing hormone (GnRH) agonists: cause chemical castration by suppressing production of estrogen/progesterone from ovaries and testosterone from testes; examples include goserelin, leuprolide, and triptorelin

- *Aromatase inhibitors*: block conversion of androgens to estrogens, used in postmenopausal breast cancer; examples include anastrozole, exemestane, and letrozole
- *Selective estrogen receptor modulator (SERM)*: can act like anti-estrogen in some organs but similar to estrogen in others; examples include raloxifene (used for chemoprevention in patients at high risk for breast cancer), tamoxifen (used in premenopausal breast cancer), fulvestrant, and toremifene
- *Hormone supplementation*: can induce feedback inhibition for synthesis of other hormones

  • Androgens: fluoxymesterone can be used in advanced breast cancer
  • Estrogens: diethylstilbestrol (DES) can be used in prostate cancer
  • Progestins: megestrol or medroxyprogesterone used in advanced breast, endometrial, or prostate cancer

• *Immunotherapy*: harnesses body's own immune system to attack cancer cells

- *Adoptive T-cell transfer*: boosts body's T cells by isolating T cells in the patient that are most active against cancer antigens and/or modifying genes to make T cells attack cancer cells, proliferating large number of T cells in vitro, and then delivering modified T cells back to patient
- *Bacille Calmette-Guérin (BCG) vaccine*: activates immune system, used in bladder cancer
- *Cytokines*: regulate and mediate immune responses and inflammation

  • Interferons: IFN-α activates natural killer (NK) cells and dendritic cells, used in melanoma, Kaposi's sarcoma, hematological cancers, renal cell, and carcinoid
  • Interleukins: IL-2 stimulates T-cell proliferation, NK cells, and B-cell antibody production, used in metastatic renal cell cancer and melanoma

- *Monoclonal antibodies (Mab)*: bind to specific antigens to prevent tumor growth or on tumor cells to mark them for destruction by immune system (can also be referred to as targeted therapy)

  • *Checkpoint inhibitors*: most work by targeting programmed death-1 (PD-1) receptors on T cells or programmed death ligand 1 (PD-L1) on tumor cells. When PD-1 binds to PD-L1, T cells are "turned off." Checkpoint inhibitors prevent tumor cells from binding to PD-1 receptor on T cells so that an anti-tumor immune response can be elicited. Examples include:

    - Atezolizumab: blocks PD-L1, used in bladder cancer and non-small cell lung cancer
    - Avelumab: blocks PD-L1, used in gastric cancer
    - Durvalumab: targets PD-L1, used in bladder cancer
    - Nivolumab: targets PD-1 receptor, used in melanoma and non-small cell lung cancer
    - Pembrolizumab: targets PD-1 receptor, used in metastatic melanoma and NSCLC
    - Another type of checkpoint inhibitor targets CTLA-4 receptors on T cells which also act as "off switch." Example includes ipilimumab used in metastatic melanoma

  • *Epidermal growth factor receptor (EGFR) inhibitors*: work by targeting EGFR which regulates cell growth and division to prevent tumor growth. Many EGFR inhibitors are Mab but some are tyrosine kinase inhibitors (see Targeted therapy below). Examples of EGFR Mab include:

    - Cetuximab: used in head and neck cancers and metastatic colorectal cancer
    - Necitumumab: used in non-small cell lung cancer
    - Panitumumab: used in metastatic colorectal cancer

- Trastuzumab (Herceptin): specifically targets human epidermal growth factor receptor 2 (HER-2) in breast cancer

- *Vascular endothelial growth factor (VEGF) inhibitors*: work by targeting VEGF to prevent growth of new blood vessels which would allow tumor to grow. Example includes:
  - Bevacizumab (Avastin): used in cervical, colorectal, lung, kidney, ovarian, fallopian tube, and primary peritoneal cancers and glioblastoma
  - Ramucirumab: used in advanced gastric, colorectal, and non-small cell lung cancer

- Other types of Mab used in immunotherapy include:

  - Alemtuzumab: targets CD52, used in B-cell chronic lymphocytic leukemia
  - Rituximab: targets CD20 on B cells, used in non-Hodgkin lymphoma and CLL

- *Immunoconjugates*: Mab bound to radioactive molecule or chemotoxic drug. Examples include:

  - 90Y-ibritumomab tiuxetan: tiuxetan bound to ibritumomab which targets CD20 and bound to radioactive yttrium-90, used in B-cell non-Hodgkin lymphoma
  - Ado-trastuzumab emtansine: anticancer drug (DM1) bound to trastuzumab, used in metastatic HER-2 positive breast cancer
  - Brentuximab vedotin: targets CD30 attached to a chemo drug (MMAE), used in Hodgkin lymphoma and anaplastic large cell lymphoma

- *Treatment vaccines*: most are under development and target antigens found on specific cancer cells, only sipuleucel-T (Provenge) approved for use in metastatic castrate-resistant prostate cancer

- *Targeted therapy*: acts on cancer-specific targets, rather than attacking all rapidly dividing cells so should have less toxicity than traditional chemotherapy; often works by blocking cell proliferation (cytostatic) rather than killing cells (cytotoxic). Some examples of common targeted therapies include:

  - *Angiogenesis inhibitors*: see bevacizumab (in immuno-therapy) and sorafenib (blocks RAF kinase and inhibits VEGFR-2 signaling cascade, used in hepatocellular carcinoma, renal cell and thyroid cancers)
  - *EGFR inhibitors*: see cetuximab and panitumumab (in immunotherapy) and afatinib (also inhibits HER2 receptor, used in metastatic non-small cell lung cancer and being investigated for breast cancer)
  - *Signal transduction inhibitors*:

    - mTOR inhibitors: everolimus (Afinitor) used in breast, lung, pancreatic, neuroendocrine, and renal cell cancers and subependymal giant cell astrocytoma
    - Proteasome inhibitor: bortezomib used in multiple myeloma
    - Tyrosine kinase inhibitors (TKI): block cell signaling and inhibit EGFR, given orally; some examples include erlotinib (Tarceva) and gefitinib used in non-small cell lung cancer; imatinib mesylate (Gleevec) which targets BCR-ABL fusion protein, used in chronic myeloid leukemia, hematologic malignan-cies, and gastrointestinal stromal tumors (GIST); and sunitinib (Sutent) used in renal cell cancer, GIST, and carcinoid tumors

  - *Targeted proteins*:

    - *ALK* inhibitors target ALK protein which increases metastatic potential; examples include crizotinib, ceritinib, alectinib, and brigatinib
    - *BRAF* inhibitors target BRAF protein which increases metastatic potential; examples include

vemurafenib used in melanomas and dabrafenib used in lung cancer
  - CDK4/6 inhibitors

- *Radiation therapy*: used in *adjuvant* or *neoadjuvant* settings and for *palliative* treatment. Can be delivered as single dose or fractionated into several doses delivered over several sessions. Types of radiation therapy include:
  - External beam: radiation source is external and delivered to local targeted area

    - Intensity-modulated radiation therapy (IMRT): uses computer-controlled linear accelerators to deliver more precise radiation dose to specific area, helps to minimize radiation toxicity to surrounding normal tissue, mostly used to treat prostate and head and neck cancers

  - Internal: radiation source is placed inside the body either via solid source (brachytherapy, e.g., seed implant in prostate cancer) or via liquid source delivered intravenously (e.g., I-131 for thyroid cancer)

- *Surgery:* used for cancer *staging*, *curative*, and *palliative* treatment.

  - Staging: breast cancer sentinel node biopsy, ovarian cancer to assess for peritoneal studding
  - Curative: depending on size, location, and type of tumor in non-metastatic disease, margins of surgical resection

    - Debulking: when surgery is not curative but is still performed to remove as much of the bulk of tumor as possible, usually prior to receipt of adjuvant therapy (often done in ovarian cancer)

  - Palliative: for symptom management in advanced (non-curable) disease, often to treat symptoms associated with obstruction (e.g., bowel obstruction in colorectal or ovarian cancer, bronchial or esophageal obstruction in lung cancer), cord compression, instability of pain associated with bone metastases, fistula repair

- Types of surgery in addition to traditional scalpel include:
  - Cryosurgery: use of extreme cold (often liquid nitrogen) to destroy cancer cells
  - Laser: can used targeted light wavelength to minimize damage to surrounding tissue

- *Transplant*: used to cure some hematological malignancies (AML, ALL, CML, refractory Hodgkin and non-Hodgkin lymphoma, multiple myeloma, myelodysplastic syndromes) and some solid tumor malignancies (neuroblastoma, Ewing sarcoma, gliomas)

  - *Bone marrow or stem cell*: can be autologous (from patient himself/herself) or from donor (syngeneic—from identical twin—or, more commonly, allogeneic); stem cells usually harvested through peripheral blood but can also come from bone marrow or umbilical cord blood; major common complications are infection and graft-versus-host disease (GVHD). Conditioning regimens prior to transplant may vary, typically including chemotherapy and/or radiation therapy
  - *Solid organ*: liver transplant used for hepatocellular cancer

Specific Cancers

Treatment decisions are based on cancer type and stage and patient characteristics (functional status, comorbidities, age) and treatment preferences. An overview of treatments for common cancers is provided below. As treatment regimens continue to evolve, we recommend the reader review the guideline resources provided later in the chapter. Treatment of other cancers is also provided in Resources.

Breast

Treatment can involve chemotherapy, hormonal therapy, radiation, surgery, and targeted therapy.

- Chemotherapy: usually combination chemotherapy regimens (two to three drugs) based on cancer stage, type, and hormone-receptor status and patient characteristics/comorbidities; common classes used include anthracyclines, taxanes, 5-FU, cyclophosphamide, and carboplatin
- Hormonal therapy: for ER+ tumors, SERM (if premenopausal) or AI (if postmenopausal); fulvestrant in advanced cancer
- Radiation therapy: adjuvant therapy, decision to give based on stage and size of tumor
- Surgery: can be breast conserving (lumpectomy or partial mastectomy) or mastectomy, will also often include sentinel node biopsy, and may include axillary lymph node dissection
- Targeted therapy: those with HER2/neu-positive tumors can be treated with trastuzumab or kinase inhibitors

Colorectal

Treatment often involves surgery and may involve chemotherapy or immunotherapy; radiation not commonly used for colon but may be used for rectal cancer.

- Chemotherapy: different chemotherapy regimens based on cancer stage and patient characteristics; 5-FU and leucovorin, oxaliplatin, or capecitabine are common chemotherapies used
- Immunotherapy: VEGF inhibitors (e.g., bevacizumab) or EGFR inhibitors (cetuximab and panitumumab) used for advanced cancer
- Surgery: partial colectomy is mainstay of treatment of early-stage cancer

Prostate

Treatment is based on Gleason score and often involves surgery and may involve chemotherapy, hormonal therapy, and radiation.

- Active surveillance (checking PSA every 3 months) is a good option for those with Gleason score <6
- Chemotherapy: often only used for advanced stage; common chemotherapies used include docetaxel, cabazitaxel, mitoxantrone, and estramustine
- Hormonal therapy: ADT with GnRH agonists or antiandrogens, can be used with radiation therapy as initial therapy or in advanced cancer
- Immunotherapy: sipuleucel-T (Provenge) can be used in castrate-resistant metastatic cancer
- Radiation therapy: external beam or brachytherapy (seed implant) can be used as initial therapy or if there is recurrence after surgery
- Surgery: prostatectomy can be performed either open or laparoscopic (with or without robotic assistance)

Lung (Non-small Cell)

Treatment can involve chemotherapy, immunotherapy, radiation, surgery, and targeted therapy.

- Chemotherapy: usually treated with combination of two chemotherapy regimens based on cancer stage, type, and patient characteristics/comorbidities; platinum-based chemotherapy with plant alkaloid is commonly used combination
- Immunotherapy: immune checkpoint inhibitors (targeting PD-1 and PD-L1) can be used in some cases to boost body's immune response against cancer cells
- Radiation therapy: can be used as adjuvant or neoadjuvant therapy, used as palliative therapy for advanced cancer

- Surgery: can be segmentectomy (wedge resection), lobectomy, or pneumonectomy
- Targeted therapy: VEGF inhibitors used in advanced cancer; those with EFGR gene mutations can be given EGFR inhibitors (e.g., erlotinib, afatinib, gefitinib); those with *ALK* gene mutations can be treated with ALK protein inhibitors

Acute Treatment Toxicities

Toxicities are often due to drug's mechanism of action and often apply to a drug class (but not always).

- Chemotherapy's cytotoxic action targets rapidly dividing cells (a feature of almost all cancer types); therefore chemotherapy can be toxic to normal cells that are also actively multiplying (e.g., cells in the bone marrow, GI tract, and hair follicles)
- Hormonal therapy's action usually targets hormone suppression; therefore its toxic effects are seen in hormonal suppression (e.g., inducing menopausal-type symptoms due to anti-estrogen effects)
- Radiation therapy's action targets local area surrounding tumor; its toxic effects often include skin changes, fatigue, nausea/vomiting, and diarrhea (for pelvic or rectal radiation)
- Targeted therapy tries to specifically target tumor cells (e.g., tumor-specific markers or gene arrangements) to minimize toxicity to normal cells, but since many therapies target EGFR or VEGF, common toxicities affect the skin or blood vessels

Factors Affecting Toxicity

- Drug dosing and schedule
- Patient functional status and comorbidities
- Cancer type

Common Acute Toxicities by Treatment Class (Table 5.3)

TABLE 5.3 Common Acute Treatment Toxicities

Treatment	Toxicity
Chemotherapy	
Alkylating agents (in general)	Neutropenia/anemia Nausea/vomiting Infertility
Busulfan	Hepatotoxicity Pulmonary toxicity Seizure
Cyclophosphamide, ifosfamide	Hemorrhagic cystitis
Nitrosoureas (e.g., carmustine)	Pulmonary toxicity
Platinum-based agents (e.g., carboplatin, cisplatin)	Nephrotoxicity Neuropathy Ototoxicity
Antimetabolites (in general)	Neutropenia/anemia Nausea/vomiting
Adenosine deaminase inhibitor (e.g., cladribine, fludarabine)	Nephrotoxicity Neurotoxicity Hepatotoxicity
Folic acid antagonist (e.g., methotrexate, pemetrexed)	Nephrotoxicity Pneumonitis Third spacing/fluid retention
Purine antagonist (e.g., 6-MP)	Hepatotoxicity
Pyrimidine antagonist (e.g., 5-FU)	Hepatotoxicity Rash Hand/foot syndrome (5-FU, capecitabine)
Anthracyclines (e.g., doxorubicin, epirubicin, daunorubicin)	Neutropenia/anemia Nausea/vomiting Cardiomyopathy Red discoloration of body fluids (except mitoxantrone causes blue/green discoloration)

TABLE 5.3 (continued)

Treatment	Toxicity
Plant alkaloid (in general)	Neutropenia/anemia
Irinotecan, topotecan	Diarrhea Nausea/vomiting Alopecia
Taxanes (e.g., paclitaxel)	Neuropathy Hypersensitivity reaction Alopecia Mucositis
Vinca alkaloids (e.g., vincristine, vinblastine)	Neuropathy Hepatotoxicity Fatigue Nausea/vomiting Anorexia
Other	
Bleomycin	Pulmonary toxicity (pneumonitis/ pulmonary fibrosis) Mucositis Rash
Retinoids	Neutropenia Hepatotoxicity
Hormonal therapy	
Androgen deprivation therapy (in general)	Hot flashes Decreased libido
Antiandrogens (e.g., bicalutamide, flutamide)	Hepatotoxicity Galactorrhea Gynecomastia
GnRH agonists(e.g., goserelin, leuprolide)	Edema Hyperlipidemia Weight gain
Aromatase inhibitors (e.g., anastrozole, exemestane, letrozole)	Hot flashes Bone/joint pain, osteoporosis Edema Hyperlipidemia

(continued)

TABLE 5.3 (continued)

Treatment	Toxicity
Selective estrogen receptor modulator (SERM) (e.g., tamoxifen, fulvestrant)	Hot flashes Thromboembolism Increased risk of endometrial cancer Edema Mood changes
Immunotherapy	Depends on specific monoclonal antibody targeted, often neutropenia
Cytokines (e.g., IFN-α, IL-2)	Flu-like symptoms Hepatotoxicity
HER-2/neu inhibitors (e.g., trastuzumab [Herceptin])	Cardiotoxicity Diarrhea Hepatotoxicity Neuropathy
PD-1 and PD-L1 inhibitors (e.g., atezolizumab, nivolumab, pembrolizumab)	Fatigue Diarrhea Rash Immunological reactions
Targeted therapy	
Angiogenesis inhibitors (e.g., bevacizumab [Avastin], sorafenib)	Delayed wound healing Hemorrhage Thromboembolism Hypertension Proteinuria
EGFR inhibitors (e.g., cetuximab, panitumumab)	Acneiform rash Hypomagnesemia Nausea/vomiting
Signal transduction inhibitors	
mTOR inhibitors (e.g., everolimus)	Angioedema Hepatotoxicity Nephrotoxicity Mucositis

TABLE 5.3 (continued)

Treatment	Toxicity
Tyrosine kinase inhibitors (e.g., erlotinib, gefitinib, imatinib)	Neutropenia Nausea/vomiting Edema Rash
Targeted proteins	
ALK inhibitors (e.g., crizotinib, ceritinib)	Fatigue Neuropathy Nausea/vomiting Hepatotoxicity
BRAF inhibitors (e.g., vemurafenib, dabrafenib)	Development of cutaneous SCC Photosensitivity Hepatotoxicity
Radiation therapy	Skin changes (dryness, itching, burn) Hair loss Fatigue Diarrhea (pelvic or rectal radiation) Cystitis (pelvic or rectal radiation)

Common Acute Toxicities and Management (Table 5.4)

Special Populations

Children/Adolescents/Young Adults

- Need to consider fertility in treatment recommendations and decisions. This should be discussed prior to treatment but, if not discussed at that time, does not preclude assessment later in treatment course

TABLE 5.4 Acute Toxicities and Management

Acute toxicity	Common treatment causes	Management
Cognitive dysfunction	Chemo, HT	Possible use of stimulants
Dermatologic		
Alopecia	Chemotherapy, RT	Scalp cooling caps
Rash	Immunotherapy, Targeted therapy	Topical steroids or clindamycin gel
Skin dryness/itch	RT	Antihistamine
Gastrointestinal		
Anorexia[a]	Chemo, RT	Increase fluid and small higher calorie food intake
Diarrhea	RT, targeted therapy	Loperamide Octreotide (subcutaneous)
Nausea/vomiting[a]	Chemo, RT	5-HT antagonists (e.g., ondansetron) Anxiolytics (e.g., lorazepam) Dopamine antagonists (e.g., metoclopramide) NK-1 antagonists (e.g., aprepitant) Steroids Cannabinoids (e.g., dronabinol)
Oral/mucositis	Chemo RT	Saline or salt/soda mouth wash Magic mouthwash
Fatigue[a]	Chemo, HT, RT	Graded exercise Psychosocial support

TABLE 5.4 (continued)

Acute toxicity	Common treatment causes	Management
Fertility	Chemo, HT, RT	Women: egg banking Men: sperm banking
Hematologic		
Anemia	Chemo	Darbepoetin (Aranesp), Erythropoietin (Epogen), PRBC transfusion
Neutropenia	Chemo, Transplant	G-CSF (e.g., Neulasta, Neupogen)
Thrombocytopenia	Chemo	Platelet transfusion
Neuropathy	Chemo	Gabapentin, pregabalin Topical lidocaine or capsaicin Acupuncture TENS
Pain[a]	RT	Treatment depends on type: nociceptive (due to ongoing tissue injury) vs. neuropathic (due to peripheral/CNS damage) Generally, try to start with non-opioids first, opioids when needed and with plan for long-term taper if possible
Sexuality	Chemo, HT, RT	Women: vaginal lubricants, vaginal moisturizers Men: PDE-5 inhibitors Both: Psychosocial interventions for sexuality/intimacy concerns

(continued)

TABLE 5.4 (continued)

Acute toxicity	Common treatment causes	Management
Sleep disturbance	Chemo	Sleep hygiene recommendations Assess for mood disorders Referral to specialist, programs

Abbreviations: 5-HT serotonin, *G-CSF* granulocyte colony stimulating factor, *PDE-5* phosphodiesterase-5
[a]For more details on this side effect and management, please see Chap. 7

  - Can recommend banking sperm/oocytes, referral to reproductive medicine specialist for consideration of strategies to preserve fertility or assess residual fertility (and for possible clinical trials)

• Recognize that some treatments can lead to increased risk for development of second cancers and other important comorbidities later in life (cardiovascular disease, pulmonary disease)

  - Need to counsel patients with regard to importance of follow-up during and after treatment for risk-based care

Older Adults

• Performance status and overall life expectancy are critical when making treatment recommendations
• Need to understand patient's values (goals of care) to arrive at treatment decisions that are aligned with patient's goals
• Presence of social support (both functional and emotional support) during treatment may be more critical for older adults

Care of Patients with Multiple Comorbidities

- Functional status and cancer prognosis are important considerations when making treatment recommendations and decisions when patients have other serious comorbidities
- More compelling need for good communication and care coordination between primary care physicians (PCPs) and specialists to optimize care during cancer treatment
- Need to emphasize that most patients with early-stage cancer (which is often curable) will outlive cancer and die from complications due to their other chronic comorbidities, so it is important not to ignore comorbidity management during active treatment

PCP Role During Active Treatment

Though patients will be receiving treatment from an oncology team, it is important for the PCP to remain engaged in their care. Evidence suggests that patients receive more comprehensive care when both oncology and primary care are involved. Examples of ways PCPs can play an active role during cancer treatment include:

- Comorbid disease management
- Keep patients up to date with vaccinations
- Monitor for acute treatment toxicities (particularly those related to cardiovascular risk factors such as hypertension, lipids, and thromboembolism risk)
- Recognize complications of therapy and work closely with the oncology team to evaluate and manage in a timely manner
- Help guide goals of care discussions
- Help with patient engagement during active treatment:

  - Question prompt list to help guide conversations about treatment decisions

- Multiple decision aids have been developed to help guide treatment decisions and have shown efficacy with increasing patient knowledge without adversely affecting patient anxiety or decisional conflict; decision aids tend to be disease and treatment specific (e.g., surgery vs. RT for prostate cancer treatment). See Additional Resources
- Confirm that patients undergoing treatment with curative intent are given treatment summary (important for transitioning to survivorship care, see Chap. 6)

- Provide psychosocial support
- Provide caregiver support

References and Additional Resources

Cancer Staging:

- American Joint Committee on Cancer (AJCC) cancer staging manual: https://cancerstaging.org/references-tools/Pages/What-is-Cancer-Staging.aspx
- American Joint Committee on Cancer (AJCC) cancer staging resources: https://cancerstaging.org/references-tools/deskreferences/Pages/Supplementary-Material.aspx

Decision Aids:

- Trikalinos TA, Wieland LS, Adam GP, et al. Decision Aids for Cancer Screening and Treatment [Internet]. Rockville (MD): Agency for Healthcare Research and Quality (US); 2014 Dec. (Comparative Effectiveness Reviews, No. 145.) https://www.ncbi.nlm.nih.gov/books/NBK269405/#_ncbi_dlg_citbx_NBK269405

Treatment:

- National Comprehensive Cancer Network: https://www.nccn.org/professionals/
- American Cancer Society resources:

- Breast cancer: https://www.cancer.org/content/dam/CRC/PDF/Public/8581.00.pdf
- Colorectal cancer: https://www.cancer.org/content/dam/CRC/PDF/Public/8607.00.pdf
- Lung cancer: https://www.cancer.org/content/dam/CRC/PDF/Public/8706.00.pdf
- Prostate cancer: https://www.cancer.org/content/dam/CRC/PDF/Public/8796.00.pdf

Tumor Markers:

- National Cancer Institute: https://www.cancer.gov/about-cancer/diagnosis-staging/diagnosis/tumor-markers-fact-sheet

Special Populations:

- *Adolescent and Young Adults:* National Comprehensive Cancer Network Guidelines for Adolescents and Young Adults with Cancer: https://www.nccn.org/patients/guidelines/aya/files/assets/basic-html/page-1.html#

  - *Fertility issues:* http://oncofertility.northwestern.edu/

- *Older adults:* National Comprehensive Cancer Network Older Adult Oncology Guidelines: https://www.nccn.org/professionals/physician_gls/pdf/senior.pdf

Chapter 6
Cancer Survivorship

Larissa Nekhlyudov

Overview

As of 2016, there are over 15.5 million individuals who have survived or are living with cancer. It is estimated that by 2026, there will be 20.3 million cancer survivors. Cancer survivors are at risk for cancer recurrence and new cancers, and may be experiencing late and long-term effects of treatment causing significant morbidity and premature mortality. This chapter provides an overview of the key issues in caring for this growing population.

Definition

The term "cancer survivor" has been variably defined. For this overview, we will use the term to describe any individual diagnosed with cancer, from the time of initial diagnosis to the time of death. However, since this handbook is intended to be used by primary care providers, we focus on those who have completed treatment. A portion of this overview will address the needs of those who are living with advanced cancer and remain under treatment.

L. Nekhlyudov (✉)
Division of General Internal Medicine and Primary Care, Brigham and Women's Hospital, Harvard Medical School, Boston, MA, USA
e-mail: lnekhlyudov@partners.org

© Springer Nature Switzerland AG 2019   125
L. Nekhlyudov et al. (eds.), *Caring for Patients Across the Cancer Care Continuum*,
https://doi.org/10.1007/978-3-030-01896-2_6

Epidemiology

- In the 1970s there were 3 million cancer survivors in the United States (USA). This number has steadily increased since, and as of 2016 there were over 15 million in the USA and 32 million worldwide. By 2040, in the USA alone, there will be 26 million cancer survivors
- The most common cancers among US survivors are female breast (23%, 3.6 million), prostate (21%, 3.3 million), colorectal (9%, 1.5 million), gynecologic (8%, 1.3 million), and melanoma (8%, 1.2 million)
- As of 2016, 67% of cancer survivors in the USA have survived 5 years or more after diagnosis, 44% have survived at least 10 years, and 17% have survived 20 years or more
- Over 60% of survivors are aged 65 and older. By 2040, 73% of survivors will be aged 65 and older. Five percent of survivors are younger than 40
- Approximately 380,000 cancer survivors who were diagnosed between birth and 19 years are currently alive

Care for Cancer Survivors

Cancer survivors face unique challenges following cancer treatment. Key areas of focus for caring for cancer survivors include the following: (1) surveillance for recurrences; (2) screening for primary new cancers; (3) genetic testing; (4) evaluation and management of physical long-term and late effects of treatment; (5) evaluation and management of psychosocial effects; (6) health promotion, disease prevention, and chronic disease management; and (7) communication and care coordination. These areas are further defined below.

Surveillance for Recurrences

This area of survivorship care focuses on detecting recurrences early. For most cancers, this includes taking a careful history and conducting a clinical examination. Laboratory testing, imaging, and other procedural recommendations vary by cancer type.

Screening for New Primary Cancers

This area of survivorship care focuses on screening for new cancers that may be related to the treatment of the initial malignancy (i.e., chemotherapy and/or radiation) or to underlying risk factors (i.e., genetics, environment, lifestyle, etc.).

Genetic Testing

This area of cancer survivorship care focuses on the assessment for possible hereditary factors that may have contributed to the initial cancer and may be associated with other cancers in the survivor and/or family members.

Evaluation and Management of Physical Long-Term and Late Effects of Treatment

This area of cancer survivorship care focuses on physical long-term (start at time of treatment) or late (start months to years after treatment) effects of treatment. The risk for such effects typically depends on the type of treatment (surgery, radiation, chemotherapy, hormonal therapy, and/ or immunotherapy/targeted therapy), duration, and dose of treatment, among other factors. Examples of such effects are outlined in Boxes 6.1 and 6.2 and in Figs. 6.1 and 6.2. For an overview of management recommendations, refer to Table 6.1.

Box 6.1 Examples of Chemotherapy-Related Long-Term and Late Effects

- Cardiac dysfunction (doxorubicin, daunorubicin, trastuzumab)
- Pulmonary fibrosis (bleomycin)
- Neuropathy (vincristine, vinblastine, paclitaxel, docetaxel, oxaliplatin, cisplatin)
- Hearing loss (cisplatin or other platinum-based agents)
- Renal/bladder dysfunction (cisplatin, cyclophosphamide)
- Premature menopause, infertility (cyclophosphamide, nitrogen mustard, or other alkylators)

Box 6.2 Examples of Surgery-Related Long-Term and Late Effects

- Lymphedema
- Pain
- Functional limitations
- Sexual dysfunction
- Body image
- Infertility
- Ostomy-related effects (both psychosocial and physical)
- Post-splenectomy infections

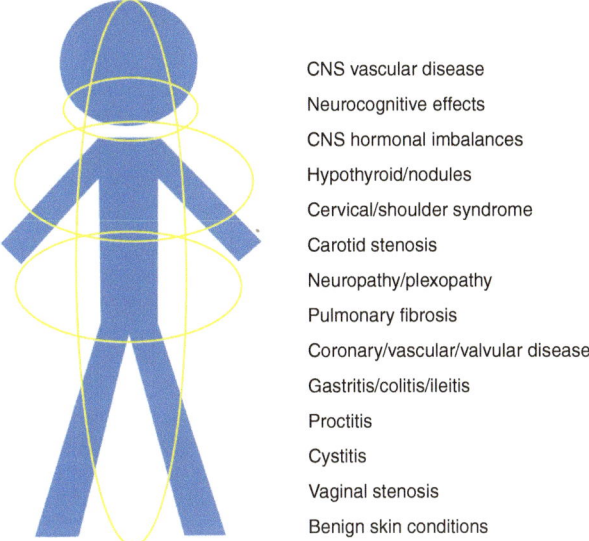

CNS vascular disease
Neurocognitive effects
CNS hormonal imbalances
Hypothyroid/nodules
Cervical/shoulder syndrome
Carotid stenosis
Neuropathy/plexopathy
Pulmonary fibrosis
Coronary/vascular/valvular disease
Gastritis/colitis/ileitis
Proctitis
Cystitis
Vaginal stenosis
Benign skin conditions

FIGURE 6.1 Secondary non-cancer effects associated with radiation. Circles represent fields of radiation

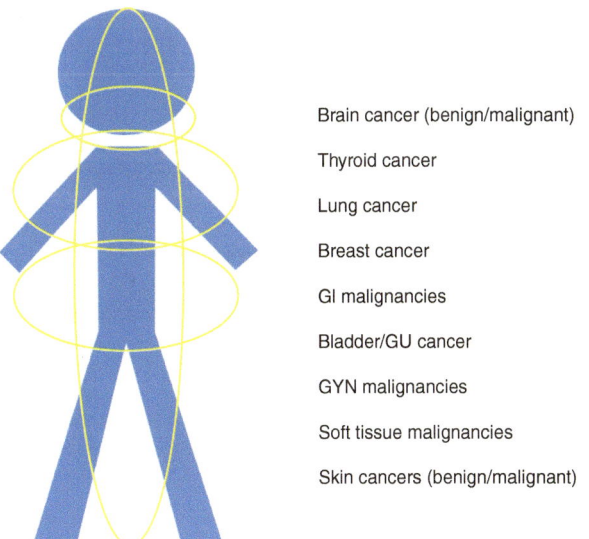

Brain cancer (benign/malignant)
Thyroid cancer
Lung cancer
Breast cancer
GI malignancies
Bladder/GU cancer
GYN malignancies
Soft tissue malignancies
Skin cancers (benign/malignant)

FIGURE 6.2 Subsequent cancers associated with radiation. Circles represent fields of radiation

Evaluation and Management of Psychosocial Effects

This area of cancer survivorship care focuses on nonphysical effects of the cancer diagnosis and treatment such as depression, anxiety, and fear of recurrences; body image, sexual health, and relationship issues; as well as financial, educational, and employment concerns. PCPs should acknowledge the impact of cancer on family and friends and provide support as needed. For an overview of management recommendations (see Table 6.1).

TABLE 6.1 Strategies for management of selected late and long-term effects following cancer treatment

Anxiety, depression, fear of recurrences	Consider physiological or other psychological etiologies[a]
	Validation
	Social support network, physical activity, nutrition
	Referral for cognitive behavioral therapy, medications
Vasomotor symptoms	Females
	Vaginal symptoms – moisturizers, lubricants, estrogen if not contraindicated, consider testosterone, referral
	Hot flashes – exercise, acupuncture, cognitive behavioral therapy, consider serotonin reuptake inhibitors (SSRIs), serotonin-norepinephrine reuptake inhibitors (SNRIs), venlafaxine, or gabapentin
	Males – venlafaxine or gabapentin may be considered for men on androgen deprivation therapy
Sleep disturbance	Consider physiological, psychological etiologies[a]
	Sleep diary, sleep hygiene, relaxation, meditation, exercise
	Referral for therapy
	Medication management

TABLE 6.1 (continued)

Sexual dysfunction	Consider physiological, psychological etiologies[a] Females – consider moisturizers, lubricants, use of dilators and vibrators, referral for pelvic physical therapy and other management options Males – consider testosterone, phosphodiesterase type 5(PDE5) inhibitors, referral for therapy and other management options
Cognitive/ memory effects	Consider physiological, psychological etiologies[a] Validation, neurocognitive evaluation, physical activity
Fatigue	Consider physiological, psychological etiologies[a] Physical activity, referral to cognitive behavioral therapy, consider medications such as stimulants
Pain	Consider physiological, psychological etiologies[a] Consider type of pain (neuropathic, chronic, myalgias, skeletal, myofascial, lymphedema, postradiation) Strategies may vary based on type of pain and may include exercise, massage, physical therapy, cognitive behavioral therapy, TENS, and medications. Avoid chronic narcotics if possible

[a]PCPs need to take a careful history, perform a physical examination, and consider additional testing to rule out conditions such as sleep apnea, thyroid dysfunction, anemia, vitamin deficiencies, and others. Psychological symptoms need to be evaluated and appropriately diagnosed.

Health Promotion, Disease Prevention, and Chronic Disease Management

- For all cancer survivors, PCPs should encourage a healthy lifestyle, including physical activity, healthy diet, smoking cessation, and limited use of alcohol. This is of particular importance for survivors of cancers that are more closely linked with lifestyle risk factors, for example, head and neck

cancers and lung cancers. Box 6.3 summarizes the recommendations for healthy lifestyles for cancer survivors
- Further, PCPs should be aware that cancer survivors are at an increased risk of late effects when there are co-existent comorbid medical conditions such as cardiovascular disease, hypertension, diabetes, or obesity. Counseling about and management of chronic medical conditions is of critical importance
- Lastly, PCPs should be aware of vaccination recommendations for cancer survivors. These are summarized in Box 6.4

Box 6.3 Healthy Lifestyle Recommendations
- Achieve and stay at a healthy weight
- Aim for 150 min of activity per week
- Strength training at least twice per week
- Minimize alcohol intake (limit to one drink per day for females, two for males)
- Limit red meat and avoid processed meat
- Plant-based diet
- Limit intake of simple sugars
- Minimize tobacco products
- Practice sun safety
- Dietary supplements not recommended, aim to get nutrients from food

Box 6.4 Vaccination Recommendations
- Vaccination prior to treatment onset if at all possible
- Survivors who are not considered immuno compromised:
  - Follow CDC recommendations for inactivated vaccines such as pneumonia (PCV13/PPSV-23), influenza, (inactivated), tetanus/Tdap, and HPV
  - Follow CDC recommendations for live vaccines avoid live vaccines for at least 3 months after treatment and consider input from appropriate specialist

- Survivors who are asplenic:

  - Follow CDC recommendations including influenza, pneumonia, meningococcal vaccination, and HIB if not administered in the past. Shingles vaccine considered safe

- Survivors who may be immunocompromised (i.e., ongoing chemotherapy, receiving monoclonal antibodies or checkpoint inhibitors, radiation, chronic leukemias, and lymphomas):

  - No live vaccinations should be administered
  - May not mount an adequate response to attenuated vaccines

- Survivors post bone marrow transplant with graft-versus-host disease:
  - No live vaccinations

Source: NCCN Guidelines Version 2.2017 – Survivorship

Communication and Care Coordination

- As cancer survivors may have ongoing care from member(s) of their oncology team, ongoing communication among the team members and the PCP is needed. This can assure that there is a common understanding of the disease prognosis, follow-up recommendations, late and long-term effects, and other aspects of cancer survivorship care outlined.
- Survivorship care plan is a record that may be used to promote PCP's understanding of the cancer diagnosis, treatment, and recommended follow-up. This document should be provided by the oncology team to all patients who are concluding active cancer treatment. The survivorship care plan must provide information about the type of cancer and treatment provided, possible late and long-term effects, and recommendations for surveillance and follow-up for these effects.

Survivorship Care Recommendations

In the following section, we outline the recommendations for selected groups of cancers. Recommendations for other cancers may be found in the Resources for Additional Learning.

Breast Cancer

Epidemiology

- Approximately 3.5 million women survivors of invasive breast cancer in the USA as of January 2016
- 19% of survivors are aged 50–59, 27% are 60–69, and 45% are 70 and older

Survivorship Care Recommendations

Surveillance for recurrences

- History and clinical examination every 3–6 months for the first 3 years after primary treatment, followed by 6–12 months for the next 2 years, and then annually
- Yearly mammography
- The following testing is not routinely recommended for most breast cancer survivors: breast MRI, laboratory testing (including liver function testing and tumor markers), and additional imaging (including chest X-ray, CT scan, and others)

Screening for new primary cancers

- Routine screening based on age – unless prior high-risk category (such as genetic mutation or radiation prior to breast cancer)

Genetic testing

- Refer women with a strong family history of cancer (including breast, colon, endometrial cancers, as well as sarcomas and brain cancers) as well as women younger than 60 with triple negative breast cancer

Evaluation and management of physical long-term and late effects of treatment

- *Lymphedema* – most commonly due to axillary lymph node dissection, less likely with sentinel node biopsy. Early recognition of lymphedema and referral to a specialized physical therapy can improve outcomes. Restricting exercise using the affected arm is no longer contraindicated
- *Cardiotoxicity* – for example, cardiomyopathy may be due to cardiotoxic chemotherapy, such as doxorubicin and trastuzumab; radiation may also contribute to cardiotoxicity leading to restrictive, valvular, and ischemic heart disease. The benefits of screening asymptomatic patients with echocardiogram (including timing and frequency) are not clear, though may be considered. Early recognition of symptoms and intervention and management as needed. Further, it is important to screen and manage conditions known to impact cardiovascular outcomes, such as hypertension, diabetes, and hyperlipidemia
- *Bone health* – may be related to early menopause and use of aromatase inhibitors. Monitoring with bone mineral density testing may be indicated. Patients should be encouraged to exercise, take calcium/vitamin D, and undergo treatment with bisphosphonates if appropriate
- *Pain and neuropathy* – may be due to surgical treatment such as mastectomy or lymphedema but also related to chemotherapy agents, including taxanes. Duloxetine may be effective for neuropathic pain. Acupuncture may be considered
- *Infertility and premature menopause/hot flashes* – may be due to chemotherapy agents, such as cyclophosphamide, as well as GnRH (gonadotropin-releasing hormone) ovarian ablation in pre- and perimenopausal women. Referral for specialty care (reproductive endocrinology) for fertility options is recommended.

Symptoms of early menopause may be responsive to exercise, selective serotonin-norepinephrine reuptake inhibitors (SNRIs), selective serotonin reuptake inhibitors (SSRIs), and gabapentin

Evaluation and management of psychosocial effects

- *Body image* – may be related to mastectomy, hair changes, and weight gain. Discuss breast prostheses, wig fitting, etc., lifestyle changes, and referral to mental health provider
- *Sexual health* – vaginal dryness may be due to early menopause as well as psychological effects. Offer non-hormonal, water-based lubricants and moisturizers. Refer for specialized sex therapy, if possible, to a provider with expertise in cancer survivorship
- *Cognitive impairment* – often referred to as "chemo brain" – this is now thought to be a valid long-term effect of treatment. Refer for neuropsychiatric evaluation, cognitive therapy. Agents such as methylphenidate, donepezil, and modafinil may be of benefit, but not currently FDA approved for this indication
- *Fear of recurrences, anxiety, and depression* – commonly observed. Encourage lifestyle interventions (e.g. exercise, yoga). Consider cognitive behavioral therapy, psychotherapy, and medical management
- *Fatigue* – assess for other etiologies (such as anemia, thyroid dysfunction, sleep apnea). Encourage lifestyle interventions (e.g. exercise, yoga). Consider cognitive behavioral therapy, psychotherapy, and medical management
- *Sleep disturbances* – assess for physical causes (such as sleep apnea, thyroid conditions), address psychological symptoms, ask patients to maintain a sleep diary, counsel on sleep hygiene, and refer to specialized program or provider
- *Financial toxicity, work, and school concerns* – patients may not disclose concerns, providers should assess and refer to available resources

Colorectal Cancer

Epidemiology

- Approximately 1.4 million survivors of colorectal cancer in the USA as of January 2016
- 13% of survivors are aged 50–59, 21% aged 60–69, and 61% aged 70 and older

Survivorship Care Recommendations

Surveillance for recurrences

- History and clinical examination every 3–6 months for the first 1–2 years, then every 6 months in years 3–5, followed by annually
- CEA every 3–6 months for the first 1–2 years, then every 6 months until year 5
- Colonoscopy in 1 year, then every 3 years (unless advanced adenoma) for 3 occurrences, then every 5 years
- Chest/abdominal/pelvic CT scan every 12 months (stages I–II if considered to be at high risk for recurrences and stage III) if additional treatment would be considered
- Routine blood tests such as blood counts, liver enzymes *not* recommended
- After 5 years, CEA and CT scans are *not* recommended

Screening for new primary cancers

- Routine age-based screening, unless genetic mutation as below

Genetic testing

- Patients with suspected familial syndromes, such as Lynch (HNPCC) or familial adenomatous polyposis (FAP), should be referred for genetics evaluation

Evaluation and management of physical long-term and late effects of treatment

- *Bowel dysfunction* – may be related to surgery, radiation therapy, and possibly chemotherapy. May consist of frequency, urgency, and incontinence, among others. With abdominal pain, must consider possible adhesions. Target interventions to suspected etiology. Consider pelvic physical therapy, anti-diarrheal medications, and dietary changes (avoid raw food, use symptom diaries, consider probiotics and low-fat diet). Biofeedback may be of benefit
- *Urinary/bladder symptoms* – these may be related to surgery, radiation, or chemotherapy. Symptoms may include urge, flow, and stress incontinence. Consider pelvic physical therapy, medications, and referral to urology. Persistent hematuria should be evaluated
- *Ostomy-related effects* – bowel resection may result in permanent ostomy. Specialized providers to offer guidance and expedited management of complications

Evaluation and management of psychosocial effects

- *Sexual health* – pelvic radiation poses a higher risk of sexual dysfunction, especially among women and those with rectal cancer. Offer non-hormonal, water-based lubricants and moisturizers. Men have erectile dysfunction that may benefit from early use of oral phosphodiesterace-5 inhibitors. Refer for specialized therapy
- *Cognitive impairment* – see discussion in Breast Cancer
- *Fear of recurrences, anxiety, and depression* – see discussion in Breast Cancer
- *Fatigue* – see discussion in Breast Cancer
- *Financial toxicity, work, and school concerns* – assess and refer to available resources

Prostate Cancer

Epidemiology

- Approximately 3.3 million survivors of prostate cancer in the USA as of January 2016
- 9% of survivors are aged 50–59, 28% are 60–69, and 62% are 70 and older

Survivorship Care Recommendation

Surveillance for recurrences

- PSA every 6–12 months for the first 5 years, then annually, if not done by specialist
- DRE – if not done by specialist

Screening for new primary cancers

- Routine age-based screening, unless genetic predisposition

Genetic testing

- Conduct careful review of family history
- Referral of survivors with early-onset prostate cancer and those with strong family history of breast, ovarian, and prostate cancer

Evaluation and management of physical long-term and late effects of treatment

- *Urinary symptoms* – symptoms may be due to surgery and/or radiation (external beam or brachytherapy) and include stress incontinence, urgency, frequency, dribbling, nocturia, urethral stricture, and hematuria. Careful evaluation of symptoms and management with medications, as well as pelvic therapy

- *Sexual dysfunction* – may be due to surgery, radiation (external beam or brachytherapy), and/or androgen deprivation therapy; symptoms include erectile dysfunction, lack of ejaculation, decreased semen, changes in orgasm, and penile shortening. Men with erectile dysfunction that may benefit from oral phosphodiesterace-5 inhibitors. Refer for specialized therapy
- *Bowel dysfunction* – symptoms may be due to surgery and/or radiation (external beam or brachytherapy), includes fecal urgency, frequency, incontinence, rectal inflammation, rectal pain, and blood in stool. Careful evaluation of symptoms. Symptomatic relief with anti-diarrheals, pelvic physical therapy
- *Vasomotor symptoms* – androgen deprivation may lead to a number of symptoms including hot flashes, weight gain, and gynecomastia. Symptoms may be treated with SNRIs and gabapentin. Gynecomastia may be treated with localized radiation therapy, surgery, or tamoxifen
- *Endocrine/metabolic changes* – androgen deprivation may lead to metabolic syndrome (including obesity, diabetes, and hyperlipidemia), cardiovascular disease, and osteoporosis. Careful monitoring and management is needed

Evaluation and management of psychosocial effects

- *Cognitive impairment* – see discussion in Breast Cancer
- *Fear of recurrences, anxiety, and depression* – see discussion in Breast Cancer. Such symptoms may be more pronounced among prostate cancer survivors in active surveillance
- *Fatigue* – see discussion in Breast Cancer
- *Financial toxicity, work, and school concerns* – assess and refer to available resources

Head and Neck Cancers

Epidemiology

- Approximately 436,000 survivors of head and neck cancers in the USA
- Cancers include those of the oral cavity, larynx, tongue, lip, pharynx, salivary glands, nasal and paranasal sinuses, and nasopharynx

Survivorship Care Recommendations

Surveillance for recurrences

- History and physical examination every 1–3 months for the first year, every 2–6 months in the second year, every 4–8 months in years 3–5, and annually after 5 years
- Additional imaging or other surveillance procedures should be coordinated with the oncology specialist
- As these survivors are at risk for recurrence, it is important to counsel patients regarding any possible suggestive symptoms. These may include any new lesions that do not heal, persistent nasal obstruction, frequent nose bleeds, difficulty swallowing, and unexplained weight loss, among others

Screening for new primary cancers

- Survivors of head and neck cancers at elevated risk for cancers, typically related to smoking in the head and neck, as well as esophageal and lung cancers
- Consider CT lung cancer screening (especially if risk factors such as smoking are present). Screening endoscopy is not routinely recommended, but may be considered for those risk factors such as smoking, alcohol, and radiation therapy. Close monitoring for symptoms and timely evaluation are recommended

Genetic testing

- No routine genetic evaluation recommended. Careful intake of family history

Evaluation and management of physical long-term and late effects of treatment

- *Musculoskeletal* – cervical dystonia, muscle spasms, spinal accessory nerve palsy, shoulder dysfunction, and lymphedema may occur following surgery or radiation. Evaluation of symptoms and referral to specialized physical therapy are important
- *Oral/dental* – trismus, dental caries, periodontitis, oral infections, candidiasis, xerostomia, and altered or loss of taste require evaluation and referral for specialty care
- *Osteonecrosis* – rapid evaluation and referral for treatment
- *Hearing* – complications including hearing loss, tinnitus, and vestibular neuropathy may occur due to radiation, chemotherapy, and surgery. Evaluation and appropriate management
- *Speech* – evaluation and referral to therapy
- *Gastroesophageal* – dysphagia, candidiasis, and weight loss require evaluation and management. Important to also assess for possible evidence of recurrence or second malignancies
- *Thyroid* – evaluation for hypothyroidism, nodules, and malignancies that may occur in the field of radiation. Yearly physical examination and thyroid laboratory testing is recommended
- *Carotid disease* – evaluation for stenosis may be considered if the neck is involved in the field of radiation

Evaluation and management of psychosocial effects

- *Cognitive impairment* – head and neck cancer survivors, particularly those treated with radiation therapy, are at higher risk for cognitive impairment. Need to differentiate from possible speech impairment, depression, or other conditions that may arise in this group of survivors. Neurocognitive evaluation may be considered

- *Fear of recurrences, anxiety, and depression* – see discussion in Breast Cancer
- *Fatigue* – see discussion in Breast Cancer
- *Sleep disturbance* – including sleep apnea may occur related to treatment
- *Body image* – may be of particular concern for head and neck survivors due to complications involving oral health, distortion of facial features, and others
- *Financial toxicity, work, and school concerns* – assess and refer to available resources

Lymphoma and Leukemia

Epidemiology

- Approximately 408,000 survivors in the USA as of January 2016
- These include leukemias (acute myelogenous leukemia, acute lymphocytic leukemia, chronic myelogenous leukemia, and chronic lymphocytic leukemia) and lymphomas (Hodgkin lymphoma and non-Hodgkin lymphoma such as diffuse large B-cell and follicular lymphoma)

Survivorship Care Recommendations

Surveillance for recurrences

- Recommendations may vary and typically include monitoring of history and physical examinations, monitoring of blood work, and imaging. See Resources for specific information

Screening for new primary cancers

- Routine age- and risk factor-based screening recommendations apply

Genetic testing

- No routine genetic evaluation recommended; however, may be warranted based on careful intake of family history

Evaluation and management of physical long-term and late effects of treatment

- *Varies by cancer treatment provided, which may include:*
  - *Chemotherapy* agents may be used including doxorubicin, vincristine, and cyclophosphamide, among others. These may be associated with late effects such as cardiac dysfunction, neurotoxicity, and second cancers (see Box 6.1)
  - *Radiation therapy* to the brain for acute leukemia, chest, mantle, or other fields for Hodgkin and non-Hodgkin lymphoma (see Figs. 6.1 and 6.2)

Evaluation and management of psychosocial effects

- *Cognitive impairment* – see discussion in Breast Cancer
- *Fear of recurrences, anxiety, and depression* – see discussion in Breast Cancer
- *Fatigue* – see discussion in Breast Cancer
- *Financial toxicity, work, and school concerns* – assess and refer to available resources

Gynecological Cancers

Epidemiology

- Approximately 760,000 survivors of uterine cancers and 235,200 ovarian cancers in the USA as of January 2016

Survivorship Care Recommendations

Surveillance for recurrences

- *Endometrial cancer* – history and physical examination every 3–6 months, extending to yearly by 5 years' posttreatment, and imaging may be indicated. See Resources for specific recommendations and/or guidelines

- *Ovarian cancer* – history and physical examination every 3–6 months, extending to yearly by 5 years' posttreatment; CA-125 may be considered, and imaging may be indicated. See Resources for specific recommendations and/or guidelines
- *Cervical, vulvar, and vaginal cancer* – history and physical examination every 3–6 months, extending to yearly by 5 years' posttreatment; imaging may be indicated. See Resources for specific recommendations and/or guidelines
- *Sarcomas* – these may include endometrial stromal sarcoma, undifferentiated uterine sarcoma, and uterine leiomyosarcoma, which may be more likely to recur and have distant metastases. Similar recommendations as endometrial but with greater consideration for imaging of the chest, abdomen, and pelvis. Endometrial stromal tumors may be more indolent but can recur late. Careful monitoring suggested
- *Malignant germ cell tumors* – history and physical examination every 3–6 months, extending over time, monitoring of tumor markers including alpha-fetoprotein (AFP) or human chorionic gonadotropin (hCG), most helpful if elevated at baseline

Screening for new primary cancers

- Routine age-based cancer screening, unless known or suspected genetic mutation

Genetic testing

- Genetic evaluation is recommended for ovarian, endometrial, and possibly sarcoma survivors

Evaluation and management of physical long-term and late effects of treatment

- Varies depending on cancer treatment provided, including extent of surgery, use of chemotherapy and/or radiation therapy (see Boxes 6.1 and 6.2 and Figs. 6.1 and 6.2)

- Sexual side effects occur including pain, vaginal dryness, and lack of libido – early recognition and referral to pelvic physical therapy, sex therapy

Evaluation and management of psychosocial effects

- *Fear of recurrences, anxiety, and depression* – see discussion in Breast Cancer
- *Fatigue* – see discussion in Breast Cancer
- *Financial toxicity, work, and school concerns* – assess and refer to available resources

Bladder Cancer

Epidemiology

Approximately 766,000 survivors of bladder cancer in the USA as of January 2016.

Survivorship Care Recommendations

Surveillance for recurrences

- Variable based on cancer stage and treatment and may include history/physical examinations, urine testing, cystoscopy, and other imaging

Screening for new primary cancers

- Patients with bladder cancer may be at risk for other cancers that may be related to smoking. Close monitoring for new symptoms and evaluation may be advised

Genetic testing

- Generally not recommended, but careful assessment of family history is needed

Evaluation and management of physical long-term and late effects of treatment

- *Urinary symptoms* – survivors treated with cystectomy and those who had pelvic radiation may have long-term urinary complications that should be assessed and managed (e.g. with medications, pelvic floor physical therapy, behavioral therapy)
- *Neurotoxicity* – chemotherapy for bladder cancer may include agents such as cisplatin, carboplatin, paclitaxel, and docetaxel, which are associated with nerve damage including hearing loss and peripheral neuropathy
- *Bowel dysfunction* – radiation to the pelvis may result in bowel dysfunction such as diarrhea and fecal incontinence, among others

Evaluation and management of psychosocial effects

- *Body image and sexual concerns* – may be experienced by those with cystostomy. Psychological support and referral to appropriate specialists are advised
- *Fear of recurrences, anxiety, and depression* – see discussion in Breast Cancer
- *Fatigue and sleep disturbance* – see discussion in Breast Cancer
- *Financial toxicity, work, and school concerns* – assess and refer to available resources

Lung Cancer

Epidemiology

- Approximately 526,000 survivors of lung cancer in the USA as of January 2016
- Lung cancer includes small cell and non-small cell (adenocarcinoma, squamous cell or epidermoid carcinoma, and large-cell carcinoma)

Survivorship Care Recommendations

Surveillance for recurrences

- Recommendations vary with focus on history and physical examination and imaging

Screening for new primary cancers

- Routine age-related screening but with attention given to other cancers that may be related to lifestyle risk factors, particularly smoking

Genetic testing

- No specific recommendations, but careful assessment of family history is needed

Evaluation and management of physical long-term and late effects of treatment

- *Dyspnea/pulmonary symptoms* – may occur after surgical resection and/or radiation
- *Neurotoxicity* – chemotherapy agents used to treat lung cancer are associated with late effects that may include nerve damage, such as hearing loss and peripheral neuropathy
- *Autoimmune complications* – immunotherapy – newer agents used to treat lung cancer have common side effects such as fatigue, nausea, constipation, diarrhea, and skin rash, but severe effects on the immune system may occur (leading to autoimmune responses). As these are new drugs, information on long-term effects of these agents is also insufficient

Evaluation and management of psychosocial effects

- *Cognitive impairment* – see discussion in Breast Cancer
- *Fear of recurrences, anxiety, and depression* – see discussion in Breast Cancer
- *Fatigue/sleep disturbance* – see discussion in Breast Cancer
- *Financial toxicity, work, and school concerns* – assess and refer to available resources

Thyroid Cancer

Epidemiology

- Approximately 805,000 survivors of thyroid cancer living in the USA as of January 2016
- Cancers are papillary, medullary, or anaplastic

Survivorship Care Recommendations

Surveillance for recurrences

- Varies based on assessment for risk of recurrences, generally involves history and physical examination, monitoring of tumor markers (thyroglobulin and thyroglobulin antibodies), and thyroid ultrasound
- Monitoring and management of thyroid function is needed. The level of TSH (thyroid-stimulating hormone) suppression varies based on risk of recurrence, with very low TSH recommended in high-risk individuals

Screening for new primary cancers

- Routine-based cancer screening, but assessment of family history is needed
- Radioactive iodine has been associated with risk of leukemia

Genetic testing

- Generally referral not advised, but important to take careful family history

Evaluation and management of physical long-term and late effects of treatment

- Survivors may be at risk for cardiac arrhythmias, possibly related to over-suppression
- Potential effects on reproductive function have been reported

Evaluation and management of psychosocial effects

- *Fear of recurrences, anxiety, and depression* – see discussion in Breast Cancer
- *Fatigue and sleep disturbance* – see discussion in Breast Cancer
- *Financial toxicity, work, and school concerns* – appears less common in thyroid cancer survivors

Melanoma

Epidemiology

- Approximately 1.2 million melanoma survivors are living in the USA as of January 2016

Survivorship Care Recommendations

Surveillance for recurrences

- Routine history and physical examinations, including skin and lymph node. Imaging may be advised for more advanced stages

Screening for new primary cancers

- Skin examinations for other melanomas, basal cell, or squamous cell carcinomas

Genetic testing

- Generally not recommended, but careful assessment of family history is needed

Evaluation and management of physical long-term and late effects of treatment

- Pain – mainly due to surgical resection
- *Neurotoxicity* – chemotherapy agents vary and may include those leading to nerve damage, such as hearing loss and peripheral neuropathy

- *Autoimmune effects* – immunotherapy – as noted in the Lung Cancer section, are associated with rare autoimmune complications that typically occur during treatment. Long-term effects are not yet known

Evaluation and management of psychosocial effects

- *Body image* – may be an issue for those with extensive surgical resection or if resection involved the face
- *Fear of recurrences, anxiety, and depression* – see discussion in Breast Cancer
- *Fatigue and sleep disturbance* – see discussion in Breast Cancer
- *Financial toxicity, work, and school concerns* – appears less common in melanoma survivors

Specific Patient Population Considerations

Bone Marrow Transplantation

Survivorship Care Recommendations

- Risk of new cancers and screening depend on underlying patient factors as well as treatment recommendations exposures such as chemotherapy (type, dose, and duration) and radiation therapy (often full body radiation is given in preparation for allogeneic bone marrow transplant)
- Type and extent of long-term and late effects depend on cancer type and treatment exposures. Bone marrow transplant survivors may be at risk for effects in all systems. Careful history, examination, and monitoring needed. (See Boxes 6.1 and 6.2 and Figs. 6.1 and 6.2.)
- Chronic graft-versus-host disease may continue long-term and includes effects on the skin, oral and vaginal mucosa, gastrointestinal tract, liver, and musculoskeletal system
- Bone marrow transplant survivors are at risk for psychosocial effects as outlined above

Adult Survivors of Childhood and Adolescent Cancers

Survivorship Care Recommendations

- Surveillance for new cancers may vary based on underlying patient factors and type of treatment. Over time, it is critical to continue to assess for family history of cancers and advise genetic evaluation if concerns arise
- Type and extent of long-term and late effects depend on cancer type and treatment exposures. (See Boxes 6.1 and 6.2 and Figs. 6.1 and 6.2.)
- As described in prior sections, psychosocial effects should be assessed, managed, and monitored. Adult survivors of childhood cancers may have a number of concerns including anxiety, depression, and fear of recurrences; interpersonal relations, fertility, and sexual function; work, school, and finances; and life and healthcare transitions, among others

Advanced or Chronic Cancer

Epidemiology

- While estimates are lacking, there is a growing population of patients who are living with advanced or chronic cancer, who are in ongoing cancer treatment

Survivorship Care Recommendations

- Primary care providers play an important role in the care of such patients, along with the cancer specialist, with focus on:
  - Treatment decision-making – addressing values and preferences, discussion of goals of care, inclusion of family, among others
  - Evaluation of symptoms – survivors may be hesitant to discuss symptoms with their oncology providers due to fear that treatment may be modified or stopped

- Symptom management – offer strategies and refer to specialty care as needed
- Psychosocial support – behavioral health, cognitive therapy, medications
- Chronic disease management – addressing diabetes management, for example, may improve symptoms and cancer-specific outcomes
- Disease prevention – immunizations may be offered to reduce risk of infectious disease complications

Additional Resources

- American Cancer Society Survivorship Guidelines: https://www.asco.org/practice-guidelines/cancer-care-initiatives/prevention-survivorship/survivorship-compendium-0
- American Society of Clinical Oncology Obesity & Cancer Resources: https://www.asco.org/practice-guidelines/cancer-care-initiatives/prevention-survivorship/obesity-cancer
- American Society of Clinical Oncology Survivorship Guidelines: https://www.cancer.org/health-care-professionals/american-cancer-society-survivorship-guidelines.html
- American Society of Clinical Oncology Tobacco Cessation Tools & Resources: https://www.asco.org/practice-guidelines/cancer-care-initiatives/prevention-survivorship/tobacco-cessation-control/tobacco-cessation-tools-resources
- Be the Match Transplant Guidelines: https://bethematchclinical.org/post-transplant-care/long-term-care-guidelines/
- Cancer Care Ontario – Survivorship Guidelines: https://www.cancercareontario.ca/en/guidelines-advice/cancer-continuum/survivorship
- Children's Oncology Group Guidelines: https://childrensoncologygroup.org/index.php/survivorshipguidelines

- National Cancer Institute, Office of Cancer Survivorship: https://cancercontrol.cancer.gov/ocs/index.html
- National Comprehensive Cancer Center Guidelines: https://www.nccn.org/professionals/physician_gls/default. aspx

References

American Cancer Society. Cancer treatment & survivorship facts & figures, 2016–2017. Atlanta: American Cancer Society; 2016.

Bluethmann SM, Mariotto AB, Rowland JH: Anticipating the "Silver Tsunami": prevalence trajectories and comorbidity burden among older cancer survivors in the United States. Cancer Epidemiol Biomark Prev. 2016;25:1029–36.

Cancer Care Ontario – Survivorship Guidelines. https://www.cancercareontario.ca/en/guidelines-advice/cancer-continuum/survivorship

Centers for Disease Control and Prevention. Global cancer statistics. 2015. https://www.cdc.gov/cancer/international/statistics.htm

Chow EJ, Anderson L, Baker KS, Bhatia S, Guilcher GM, Huang JT, et al. Late effects surveillance recommendations among survivors of childhood hematopoietic cell transplantation: a Children's Oncology Group report. Biol Blood Marrow Transplant. 2016 May;22(5):782–95.

Cohen EE, LaMonte SJ, Erb NL, Beckman KL, Sadeghi N, Hutcheson KA, et al. American Cancer Society head and neck cancer survivorship care guideline. CA Cancer J Clin. 2016 May;66(3):203–39. Epub 2016 Mar 22. Review. Erratum in: CA Cancer J Clin. 2016 Jul;66(4):351.

El-Shami K, Oeffinger KC, Erb NL, Willis A, Bretsch JK, Pratt-Chapman ML, et al. American Cancer Society colorectal cancer survivorship care guidelines. CA Cancer J Clin. 2015 Nov-Dec;65(6):428–55.

Majhail NS, Rizzo JD, Lee SJ, et al. Recommended screening and preventive practices for long-term survivors after hematopoietic cell transplantation; Center for International Blood and Marrow Transplant Research (CIBMTR), American Society for Blood and Marrow Transplantation (ASBMT), European Group for Blood and Marrow Transplantation (EBMT), Asia-Pacific Blood and Marrow Transplantation Group (APBMT),

Bone Marrow Transplant Society of Australia and New Zealand (BMTSANZ), East Mediterranean Blood and Marrow Transplantation Group (EMBMT) and Sociedade Brasileira de Transplante de Medula Ossea (SBTMO). Co-published in Biol Blood Marrow Transplant. 2012;18(3):348–71; Bone Marrow Transplant. 2012;47(3):337–41; and Hematol Oncol Stem Cell Ther. 2012;5(1):1–30.

National Comprehensive Cancer Center Guidelines. https://www.nccn.org/professionals/physician_gls/default.aspx

Nekhlyudov L, Lacchetti C, Davis NB, Garvey TQ, Goldstein DP, Nunnink JC, et al. Head and neck cancer survivorship care guideline: American Society of Clinical Oncology clinical practice guideline endorsement of the American Cancer Society guideline. J Clin Oncol. 2017 May 10;35(14):1606–21.

Resnick MJ, Lacchetti C, Bergman J, Hauke RJ, Hoffman KE, Kungel TM, et al. Prostate cancer survivorship care guideline: American Society of Clinical Oncology Clinical Practice Guideline endorsement. J Clin Oncol. 2015 Mar 20;33(9):1078–85.

Rock CL, Doyle C, Demark-Wahnefried W, Meyerhardt J, Courneya KS, Schwartz AL, et al. Nutrition and physical activity guidelines for cancer survivors. CA Cancer J Clin. 2012. CA Cancer J Clin. 2013 May;63(3):215.

Runowicz CD, Leach CR, Henry NL, Henry KS, Mackey HT, Cowens-Alvarado RL, et al. American Cancer Society/American Society of Clinical Oncology breast cancer survivorship care guideline. J Clin Oncol. 2016 Feb 20;34(6):611–35.

Salani R, Khanna N, Frimer M, Bristow RE, Chen L. An update on post-treatment surveillance and diagnosis of recurrence in women with gynecologic malignancies: Society of Gynecologic Oncology (SGO) recommendations. Gynecologic Oncol. 2017;146:3–10.

Chapter 7
Palliative Care/End-of-Life Care

Linda Overholser and Allison Wolfe

Overview

This chapter will address the role of palliative care across the cancer care continuum, with emphasis on advance care planning, communication, and decision-making. It will also provide readers with management strategies for common symptoms experienced by patients at the end of life.

Palliative Care Definition

Commonly utilized is the definition from the World Health Organization: "…*an approach that improves the quality of life of patients and their families facing the problems associated with life-threatening illness, through the prevention and relief of suffering by means of early identification and impeccable*

L. Overholser (✉)
Division of General Internal Medicine, University of Colorado School of Medicine, Aurora, CO, USA
e-mail: Linda.Overholser@ucdenver.edu

A. Wolfe
Division of General Internal Medicine, University of Colorado School of Medicine, Aurora, CO, USA

© Springer Nature Switzerland AG 2019   157
L. Nekhlyudov et al. (eds.), *Caring for Patients Across the Cancer Care Continuum*,
https://doi.org/10.1007/978-3-030-01896-2_7

assessment and treatment of pain and other problems, physical, psychosocial and spiritual."

Fundamental concepts in palliative care include:

- A focus on maintaining or improving an acceptable quality of life, as defined by the patient
- The underlying diagnosis is serious but not necessarily terminal
- Support and planning should begin early in the disease trajectory
- Palliative care does not exclude life-prolonging or curative treatments
- Support should be extended to family and caregivers, including during the bereavement period
- Care should include where possible an interdisciplinary team
- Communication about goals of care should be clear and occur during all phases of care

Hospice care generally refers to care that focuses on comfort and quality of life when a disease is considered terminal.

- A condition is considered terminal when life expectancy is 6 months or less
- Does not include care with the primary goal of prolonging life
- Comorbidities can still be managed, but with the goal of providing comfort only. This may include withholding active or preventative treatment

Communication and Coordination of Care

General overview of palliative care assessments:

- Care should start with a comprehensive initial palliative care assessment
- Ongoing assessments should be repeated over time, as an individual patient's goals and preferences for care may change

- Assessments should include the participation of team members that can help to assess specific domains of care such as psychosocial, emotional, spiritual, and/or practical concerns
- Care should be coordinated with the oncology team so that information provided to the patient and family is consistent

Clear communication between the patient and healthcare team cannot be underestimated. Misperceptions about care on the part of both providers and patients can lead to:

- Seeking overly aggressive or invasive care that does not improve quality of life
- Giving up hope and limiting options for care that might be beneficial

Communication strategies that encourage patient-centered conversations about palliative care include:

- Maintaining communication with other providers to ensure that information is consistent
- Using open-ended questions to initiate conversations about goals of care or to clarify decisions being made by the patient
- Encouraging patients/caregivers to prepare specific questions ahead of time
- Validating fears, emotions, and concerns expressed by patients
- Avoiding technical jargon
- Acknowledging lack of certainty when present
- Confirming the role of family or surrogate decision-makers in care
- Assessing a patient's understanding of information discussed

Clarifying *goals of care* is more than just documenting resuscitation status or naming surrogate decision-makers. It includes gaining a thorough understanding of the preferences of the patient and their care in domains of:

- Preferences for receiving information
- Functional goals

- Goals with regard to family involvement
- Identifying specific sources of anxiety

A conversation guide that includes samples of questions to ask is included here (Fig. 7.1).

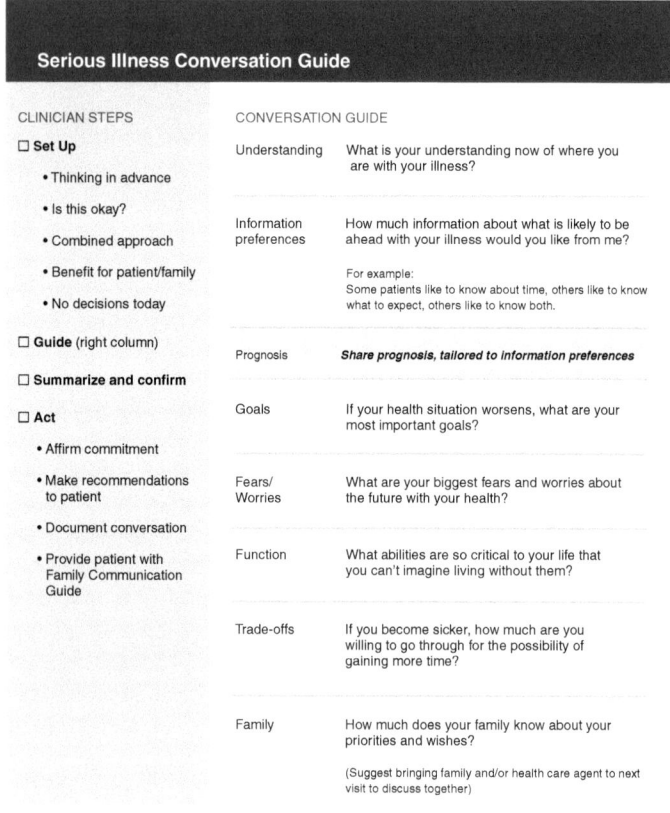

FIGURE 7.1 Sample Palliative Care Conversation Guide. © 2015–2017 Ariadne Labs: A Joint Center for Health Systems Innovation (www. ariadnelabs.org) between Brigham and Women's Hospital and the Harvard T.H. Chan School of Public Health, in collaboration with Dana-Farber Cancer Institute. Licensed under the Creative Commons Attribution-NonCommercial-ShareAlike 4.0 International License, http://creativecommons.org/licenses/by-nc-sa/4.0/ Used with permission

Patient-Centered Decision-Making

A first step in engaging in shared decision-making with any patient is to properly assess their ability (or capacity) to do so. *Capacity is not the same as competency.*

- *Capacity* describes a person's ability to make individual decisions. This is a clinical judgment; it does not require a psychiatrist or legal expertise. The presence of neurocognitive deficit or mood disorder does not necessarily render someone incapacitated to make medical decisions. The capacity to make decisions includes all of the following:
  - The ability to understand information (i.e., diagnosis, prognosis)
  - The ability to apply this information to one's own specific circumstances
  - The ability to understand the consequences of making a decision
  - The ability to indicate a choice when presented with options
- *Competency* is a broader, legal determination of which decision-making capacity is only one element

Role of Family and Caregivers

Family members are likely to be the primary source of caregiving for patients. Key concepts to consider with regard to family and other caregivers in palliative care include:

- Who participates in caregiving for a patient should be defined by the patient
- Providing support for family members is included in the working definition of palliative care
- The *National Consensus Project Clinical Practice Guidelines for Quality Palliative Care, fourth edition (2018)*, states that bereavement services and support

should be made available to families and continue for a minimum of 13 months following the death of the patient

- Family caregivers who experience stress in their role may be at increased risk themselves for morbidity and mortality

Overview of Issues/Management

Benefits of Palliative Care

Palliative care assists *patients* in numerous ways by:

- Improving patients' symptoms
- Clarifying treatment options
- Helping patients and families make difficult decisions
- Improving patients' quality of life
- Reducing hospital/emergency room visits, especially in the last days of life
- Reducing the incidence of dying as an inpatient

Palliative care can help *caregivers* by:

- Decreasing caregiver stress
- Helping to meet their needs during grieving
- Improving satisfaction with care

Palliative care can help the *healthcare system* by:

- Reducing healthcare costs
- Reducing unnecessary care

Triggers for Referral

Deciding when to consult palliative care can be difficult; however palliative care should be considered as early as possible in the treatment trajectory. The few validated screening tools have only been studied in hospitalized patients. However, in our opinion these could be extrapolated to the outpatient setting.

- CARING Criteria: Describes five indicators that identify patients appropriate for palliative care
  - The indicators are having a *C*ancer diagnosis, having greater than two *A*dmissions for a chronic illness in the last year, *R*esidence in a nursing home, *I*CU admission with multi-organ failure, and meeting two *N*on-cancer hospice *G*uidelines for an illness
  - Each individual criterion, except residence in a nursing home, was a significant independent predictor of death at 1 year
  - Screening for nursing home residence remains important as it is a proxy for poor functional status, which predicts an increased mortality risk

Delivery Models

Palliative care can be delivered in multiple ways; however, it is not available in all hospitals. In 2000, about one-quarter of hospitals with more than 50 beds had a palliative care program, and in 2015, 75% of hospitals with more than 50 beds had a palliative care program (National Palliative Care Registry 2016).

Inpatient Palliative Care Units

- Present in fewer than 10% of hospitals
- Consider if aggressive symptom management or hospital-based treatments are needed (e.g., chemotherapy or radiation therapy, wound care)
- May allow for specialized procedures, i.e., ketamine infusions for complex or intractable pain

Inpatient Palliative Care Consults

- Most of hospital-based palliative care is performed through consults

Community- or Home-Based Palliative Care

- Consider for patients who are frail and elderly or whose illness makes transportation difficult
- Example would be a nurse practitioner visiting the home once or twice a month to help with symptom management and goals of care discussions
- Can usually be delivered in nursing homes as well

Outpatient Palliative Care Clinics

- This is a new model of care and can also be delivered in nursing homes
- Appropriate for patients who can still easily travel to the clinic or who prefer not to have providers in their home

Practical Concerns

Coverage and Reimbursement

- Many private insurance plans offer coverage for palliative care under their hospice and chronic care benefits
- Medicare Part B may cover some treatments and services that provide palliation such as doctor/nurse practitioner/ social worker visits
- Medicaid may also cover some treatments and services for palliative care
- Co-pays are dependent on individuals' unique plans

Billing for Advance Care Planning

- Advance care planning (ACP), for billing, is defined as "face-to-face service between a physician or other qualified healthcare professional and a patient, family member, or surrogate in counseling and discussing advance directives, with or without completing relevant legal forms" (CPT® 2016 Professional Edition)

- The CPT codes are 99497 (covers the first 30 min of discussion) and 99498 (covers each additional 30 min). Per CPT guidelines, you can use the above codes when 1 min more than the midpoint of the code is reached (for instance, if you spend 16 min discussing ACP, you may bill with 99497)
- Completion of an advance directive is not needed to bill, but the following should be documented:
  - What was discussed
  - Patient care preferences
  - Time spent discussing ACP
  - If any family members or surrogate decision-makers were present
  - If the patient was present (the patient does not need to be present)
  - Location of service (codes may not be used for telephone visits)

ACP codes may be billed during same visit as evaluation and management codes or they can be separate. There is no limit on how often these codes can be used.

Prognostication

- Patients want detailed information about cancer prognosis, but most physicians feel poorly trained to provide it
- When prognosis is discussed, patients are more likely to complete advanced directives and less likely to desire CPR if prognosis is poor
- A multidisciplinary approach with the treating oncology team is crucial
- Discussing prognosis with patients allows them to plan and to make more informed decisions about treatment. Not doing so can lead to aggressive care at the end of life and lack of focus on symptom management/quality of life. Planning may include determining if providing care at home is feasible

The Surprise Question: Asking "Would I be surprised if this patient died in the next year?" has been shown to be a useful prognostic tool (Moss et al. 2010).

- Evidence suggests that when the answer is no, it is more predictive of 1-year mortality than age/stage/type of cancer
- Palliative care is recommended if the answer is "no"
- A "no" answer was 75% sensitive and 90% specific with a PPV of 41% and a NPV of 97% (the PPV was not high as the prevalence of death in this group was low)

Resources to help assess performance status:

- Eastern Cooperative Oncology Group Scale: http://ecog-acrin.org/resources/ecog-performance-status
- Palliative Performance Scale: https://www.mypcnow.org/blank-irr0h

Physician-Assisted Dying

Physician-assisted dying (PAD) involves a physician providing the means (a prescription) for a patient to end his or her own life at their own request, but not actually administering a drug to do so.

- PAD is not the same as withdrawal of or withholding treatment, which is considered ethical and legal in the United States (US) if that is the decision of the patient or surrogate decision-maker
- It is also distinct from voluntary euthanasia, which is illegal in the United States
- At the time of this writing, PAD is legal or not illegal in seven states/legal jurisdictions in the United States (Oregon, Washington State, Vermont, Montana, California, Colorado, and the District of Columbia), but only for adults over the age of 18

  - The legality of PAD is currently determined at a state, not federal, level
  - Medical providers need to be aware of legal status in their own state
  - Where it is legal, prognosis must be terminal
  - Waiting periods may apply

- Most requests for PAD come from individuals with cancer
- Ethical principles involved in the debate about PAD include patient autonomy, beneficence, nonmaleficence, and justice

If a request for PAD is made, some strategies could help (Spence et al. 2017):

- Being very clear about the specific request being made
- Clarifying why such a request is being made. Reasons may include fear of *anticipated* symptoms or treatment effects rather than current distress, feeling a loss of control, or feeling like a burden to loved ones
- Maximizing palliative and supportive care to manage symptoms and distress. PAD is not a substitute for palliative care
- Consultation with the oncology team, a palliative care specialist, ethicist and/or colleagues
- Assessing decision-making capacity and addressing any mental health concerns
- Ensuring that the patient is not being coerced into making the request
- Continuing to reassess patient goals of care
- Reassuring the patient that they will not be abandoned even if the PAD request is not granted

Advance Care Planning and Advance Directives

- Advanced care planning (ACP) definition: The process by which patients, families, and physicians discuss patient preferences for care, especially what they may or may not find acceptable if they have a terminal illness or irreversible condition
- May involve the completion of *advance directives*, of which several types exist:

Living Will

- Legal document describing the type of medical treatment a person would or would not want if he/she has a terminal/irreversible illness
- Delineates under what conditions life-prolonging interventions should be started, continued, or stopped
- A patient may revoke their living will at any time
- If a patient spends time in multiple states, he/she should create living wills in each state

Medical Durable Power of Attorney (MDPOA)

- Legal document in which the patient names the person who will make medical decisions for them if they lose capacity
- The MDPOA should know the patient's wishes
- The surrogate decision-maker should make decisions based on what the *patient* would decide ("substituted judgment")

The Five Wishes

- A standardized type of living will be recognized in most states
- Allows patients to name their MDPOA; describe under what conditions they would like life-prolonging treatment started, continued, or stopped; how they want to be treated; how they would like to be remembered; and what they would like done with their remains

Out-of-Hospital Do Not Resuscitate Orders

- Intended for emergency medical service teams who are required to try to resuscitate unless this form is present
- Must be signed by the patient and physician

- A bracelet or necklace may be ordered to be worn in public
- EMS teams are trained to look for these forms on the refrigerator of a patient's home if called to the home

Physician Orders of Life-Sustaining Treatment (POLST)

- For seriously ill patients, covers patients' preferences regarding CPR and level of treatment desired while alive, for example, comfort care vs selective treatment. The level of selective treatment may be quite specific such as patient would like to be hospitalized but would not want to go to the ICU. Of course, the patient could wish to have "full treatment," e.g., the patient would like ICU-level care if indicated. Also states patient's thoughts around artificial nutrition and hydration
- Should be followed in multiple settings: in hospitals, clinics, nursing homes, and the home
- Recognized in most states but can have different names

  - ACP and completion of advance directives improve concordance between patients' preferences regarding end-of-life care and the care they receive at the end of life
  - ACP discussions do not cause patients' psychosocial distress despite physicians citing this as a barrier
  - Most, but not all, states have a default surrogate decision-maker hierarchy

Symptom Management

The following section is focused on the management of more acute symptoms that may develop later in the cancer course or in those with advanced cancer who are being treated for comfort. Management of acute symptoms during active cancer treatment and late effects of cancer and its management may be found in Chaps. 5 and 6, respectively.

A useful scale to help assess common symptoms in cancer patients is the Edmonton Symptom Assessment Scale (the ESAS), which measures symptoms severity on a scale from 1 to 10 (Bruera et al. 1991).

Physical

Dyspnea

- May be described as a feeling like breathing is more rapid, that a breath does not go all the way out, having more air hunger, or a sense of suffocation
- Dyspnea may occur as a result of cancer itself (i.e., obstruction due to lung mass), cancer treatment (i.e., cardiomyopathy related to chemotherapy, surgical resection, or radiation), and comorbidities or may present as a late effect of treatment. Disease severity does not always correlate with degree of dyspnea experienced
- May be continuous, with exertion, intermittent, or acute or chronic
- Associated with decreased patient and family well-being and increased staff anxiety
- The standard for assessing dyspnea is the patient-reported experience
- Three main factors contribute to dyspnea: (1) the need for greater respiratory effort (i.e., obstruction), (2) an increase in the number of muscles required to maintain a normal workload (i.e., weakness), and (3) an increase in ventilatory needs (i.e., fever, anemia). Anatomically, obstruction, restriction, perfusion/oxygenation mismatch, and fatigue/weakness contribute to dyspnea
- *Treatment principles:* First ensure the underlying illness is medically optimized, and if so, focus on the symptom itself. Dyspnea can cause patients' spiritual and existential distress. To fully treat dyspnea, these nonphysical factors should be explored as well

- Opioids

  • Considered first-line treatment of acute dyspnea and may be considered for patients with advanced cancer especially if pain is present or for those whose primary treatment goal is comfort care
  • Thought to affect the body's response to hypercarbia and hypoxia resulting in decreased oxygen consumption
  • Modifies one's perception of dyspnea through activation of opioid receptors in the limbic system
  • Effective in the oral, parenteral, and subcutaneous forms, but nebulized opioids are not effective
  • Any type of opioid could be considered
  • Most clinicians fear respiratory depression and hastened death when using opioids in this scenario, but evidence shows this fear is unsubstantiated when opioids are appropriately titrated
  • *Please see "Pain" section on how to dose and titrate opioids*

- *Other Treatments*

  • Benzodiazepines have not been shown to improve dyspnea alone; should be considered as second- or third-line therapy in refractory dyspnea or dyspnea associated with anxiety
  • Benefits of inhaled furosemide limited to case reports
  • Supplemental oxygen therapy for comfort has not consistently shown a benefit; reserve for individuals with symptomatic hypoxemia
  • A fan blowing air across a patient's face can improve dyspnea that is related to breathlessness in those with advanced cancer
  • For patients with a good performance status, aerobic exercise (30 min of exercise a day) can help

- Catheter placement for malignant effusions resulted in improved quality of life and improvement of symptoms
- Acupuncture has had mixed results regarding benefit

Constipation

- Characterized by infrequent stools (<3 times/week or less than usual habits); stools that are small, hard, and difficult to pass; the inability to defecate at will; painful bowel movements associated with straining; unproductive urges; or sensation of incomplete evacuation
- Prevalence ranges from 23% to 70% in patients with terminal illness (Librach et al. 2010) and up to 90% of patients who are also taking opioids (Nalamachu et al. 2015)
- If present, should consider malignant bowel obstruction. If that is ruled out, constipation in cancer patients can be multifactorial and can occur as a result of cancer itself, from treatment or as a late effect. For example:

  - Medications (e.g., opioid medications, iron)
  - Decreased food/fluid/fiber intake
  - Physical (i.e., nerve impairment, pelvic surgery, or radiation)
  - Physiologic issues (e.g., electrolyte disturbances, hypercalcemia)
  - Decreased mobility (e.g., weakness, sedation)
  - Psychological (i.e., discomfort or pain with defecation)

- Even patients with anorexia should have bowel movements. Unlike other side effects of opioids, patients do not develop tolerance to constipation
- Complications of chronic constipation include rectal pain/burning, bowel obstruction, bowel rupture, and death, as well as upper gastrointestinal tract issues like gastroesophageal reflux disease (GERD)

- Can cause effects on different body systems, such as genitourinary infections secondary to urinary retention with constipation
- May decrease quality of life of the patient and caregivers
- *Treatment principles:* Goals include alleviation of pain, return of normal bowel movements, and improving associated symptoms such as nausea/vomiting

  - If opioid-induced: avoid decreasing or discontinuing opioids as this could trigger a pain crisis

    - Stool softeners and a bowel regimen should be initiated early to try to prevent constipation if opioids are used

  - *Non-pharmacologic Treatments* (may be difficult in advanced disease):

    - Maintaining adequate fluid intake
    - Adequate dietary fiber (requires adequate water intake)
    - Adequate physical activity
    - Chronic constipation that may be due to structural damage may be amenable to pelvic floor physical therapy
    - Manual evacuation may be necessary for constipation refractory to pharmacologic treatments

  - *Pharmacological Treatments*

    - Robust evidence is lacking
    - Limited level of efficacy for all laxatives

  - *Newer Treatments*

    - *Methylnaltrexone:* Approved for subcutaneous use in patients with opioid-induced constipation (OIC) not responsive to laxatives. Restricted ability to cross the blood-brain barrier, can help reverse constipation without affecting pain control. It is contraindicated in known or suspected bowel obstruction. Adverse events include nausea, flatulence, abdominal pain, and perforation (in individuals whose GI structural integrity compromised)

- *Naloxegol:* An oral opioid mu receptor antagonist, studied in OIC and non-cancer pain. Usual dose is 12.5 or 25 mg daily. Side effects include nausea, vomiting, and abdominal pain
- *Alvimopan:* Only approved for helping to resolve postoperative ileus
- *Lubiprostone:* Limited efficacy in clinical trials
- *Prucalopride:* Clinical trial efficacy data may not extrapolate to cancer and palliative care population

Nausea and Vomiting

- Nausea and vomiting may be due to underlying cancer, acute effects of radiation, and most often experienced during chemotherapy treatment. However, non-cancer-related etiologies should be considered
- History and physical examination can help to identify cause. If not identified on history and physical, consider laboratory workup to check for electrolyte imbalance, renal failure, and liver failure and to check for blood levels of medications (i.e., digoxin, phenytoin, carbamazepine, and tricyclic antidepressants)
- May lead to dehydration, electrolyte disturbances, poor nutrition, and decreased quality of life
- Affects 62% of patients with prognosis of 1–2 months and 71% of patients in last week of life
- *Treatment principles:* Include discontinuing unnecessary medications, including herbals; assessing for and treating hypercalcemia, uremia, dehydration, gastritis/GERD, and constipation

  - *Pharmacologic Treatment:* See Table 7.1 Classes of medications work on different receptors

    - If monotherapy is only partially effective, add another agent from a different class rather than rotating, as multiple receptors likely involved

TABLE 7.1 Agents to consider for specific types of nausea and vomiting

Class/name of agent	Indication
The "setrons" (i.e., ondansetron, granisetron)	Chemotherapy-induced nausea and vomiting (CINV), radiation-induced nausea and vomiting
Aprepitant (Emend)	CINV
Atypical antipsychotic (olanzapine)	CINV
Scopolamine patch	Vestibular or motion-induced
Phenothiazines (prochlorperazine, chlorpromazine, promethazine)	Promethazine: vestibular
Butyrophenones (droperidol and haloperidol)	Opioid-induced nausea/vomiting, malignant bowel obstruction
Benzamide (metoclopramide)	Gastroparesis, partial small bowel obstruction, opioid-induced nausea and vomiting
Antihistamines (hydroxyzine)	Nausea and vomiting from vestibular dysfunction
Benzodiazepines (lorazepam)	Anticipatory nausea and vomiting
Glucocorticoids (dexamethasone)	CINV, CNS involvement, gastric outlet obstruction
Cannabinoids (dronabinol)	Not recommended as first line. Reserve for intractable/refractory nausea/vomiting
Antidepressant (mirtazapine)	Consider in persistent/refractory nausea

– *Non-pharmacological Treatment*
  • Massage, foot massage shown to reduce nausea
  • Consider acupuncture, hypnosis, and cognitive behavioral therapy

- If gastric outlet obstruction or small bowel obstruction present, consider G-tube if other treatments not helping
  - *Chemotherapy-Induced Nausea and Vomiting*
    - Can be acute or delayed (begins or persists >24 h after chemo). Mediated through activation of neurotransmitters in the brain (dopamine, serotonin, substance P), as well as enterochromaffin intestinal cells. Primary treatment principle is prevention, with the use of the following agents:
      - 5-HT3 receptor antagonist + dexamethasone + aprepitant effective for highly emetogenic therapies
      - 5-HT3 receptor antagonist + dexamethasone + olanzapine effective for acute and delayed nausea/vomiting
  - *Opioid-Induced Nausea and Vomiting*
    - Mediated through brain dopamine chemoreceptors, heightened vestibular sensitivity, and/or slowed GI motility and constipation. Dexamethasone may be helpful to prevent at 10 mg/day. Once symptoms start, 5-HT3 receptor antagonists are helpful. When symptoms start, consider reducing opioid to add adjunctive therapy or trial of different opioids
    - *Radiation-induced emesis*: Occurs 30 min to 4 h after treatment and can last 2–3 days. Unclear etiology but may be mediated through irritation of brain chemoreceptor zone, damage to GI mucosa, altered smell/taste, or factors released from tumor. Preventive approach with 5-HT3 receptor antagonists +/− dexamethasone
    - If etiology unclear, consider starting with dopamine receptor antagonists or 5-HT3 and then add corticosteroids, antipsychotics, or cannabinoid if needed
    - For refractory symptoms consider inpatient admit and/or palliative care referral

Cachexia and Anorexia

- Unintentional weight loss of 5–10% of one's premorbid weight or weight loss greater than 2% when sarcopenia also present
- These symptoms are indicative of a poor prognosis; cachexia usually associated with anorexia. Tend to occur with solid tumors and in the elderly
- These may occur due to the interaction of tumor byproducts with patient cytokines, creating acute phase proteins and diminishing production of muscle protein
- Nutritional supplements, appetite stimulation usually do not reverse weight loss or loss of lean muscle mass
- Can quantify using scale such as the ESAS (as noted above)
- Patients who are obese and have sarcopenia may have poorer prognosis
- For patients with prognosis of months to years, assess for rate and severity of weight loss and screen for associated symptoms or conditions such as dysgeusia, xerostomia, mucositis, oral candidiasis, depression, early satiety, nausea/vomiting, constipation, pain, fatigue, hypogonadism, thyroid disease, and metabolic derangements
- *Treatment principles:* Include optimizing management of associated symptoms. Pharmacologic interventions may improve appetite but will not generally reverse cachexia

  – *For patients with months to years:*

    - Consider nutrition consult
    - Consider IV hydration/nutrition if within goals of care (assure MDPOA in place prior, as many states do not allow medical proxy to discontinue this)
    - May consider appetite stimulant

  – *For patients with weeks to months:*

    - Treat associated symptoms and consider appetite stimulant

- Educate patients and their families about natural course of disease
- Normalize that weight loss is common, not a sign they are "doing anything wrong"

- *For patients with days to weeks:*

  - Normalize as part of the natural course of disease/dying process
  - Reassure patient and family that patients may not feel hungry or thirsty and are not in pain from not eating/drinking
  - Educate patient/family that artificial/nutrition at this stage usually does not reverse cachexia and comes with many risks and could actually hasten death
  - Dry mouth can be sufficiently treated with good oral care
  - Withholding or withdrawing artificial nutrition/hydration is an ethically acceptable choice
  - Patients should not be forced to eat, but can be offered food

- *Megestrol (Megace):* Positive effects on appetite stimulation occur relatively quickly, but weight gain only occurs in a minority of patients and may take several weeks. Weight gain may be mostly fat/fluid and may not improve quality of life. Dosing starts at 160 mg per day, and titrate up to 400–800 mg/day. DVT, edema, and death more common; prolonged use can lead to adrenal/gonadal suppression
- *Corticosteroids:* May help improve appetite, but effect may only last on the order of weeks; consider use in patients with prognosis on this order. Common dosages: prednisone 20–40 mg daily and dexamethasone (preferred) 4–8 mg/day. Side effects include GI bleeding, oral candidiasis, and proximal myopathy
- *Dronabinol (synthetic cannabinoid):* Is FDA approved for anorexia due to AIDS and CINV, however often also used for cancer-related anorexia. Has limited effect

in patients with advanced cancer. Side effects include sedation, confusion, and perceptual disturbances

- *Mirtazapine:* An antidepressant that has been associated with weight gain, but very limited evidence in cancer
- *Artificial nutrition:* Whether via enteral or parenteral routes, usually ineffective. May delay and/or complicate transition to hospice. In advanced cancer may decrease survival and increased infection rates

Fatigue

- National Comprehensive Cancer Network definition of cancer-related fatigue: "a distressing persistent, subjective sense of physical, emotional and/or cognitive tiredness or exhaustion related to cancer or cancer treatment that is not proportional to recent activity and interferes with usual functioning"
- Most prevalent symptom in patients with cancer that may occur at diagnosis persists for months to years after treatment completion
- Etiology likely multifactorial: pain, pre-existing physical conditions, medications, psychological comorbidities, deconditioning, physiologic, or endocrine derangements
- Important to screen and rescreen over time. A single question can help: "How would you rate your fatigue on a scale from 0 to 10 over the past 7 days?"
- *Treatment principles:* No one treatment clearly superior to others

    - *Non-pharmacologic:* Strategies include exercise, though ideal type, intensity, duration unknown; psychoeducation, encouraging patients to keep diary to identify triggers and what improves symptoms; energy conservation and activity management
    - *Pharmacologic: Methylphenidate* increases levels of dopamine in the central nervous system. Has rapid onset of action, so if no benefit seen in 24–48 h, can be

quickly discontinued. Not recommended for prolonged use due to side effects (for example, decreased appetite). Dosing starts low (2.5 mg twice a day) up to 10–40 mg daily in twice daily divided dosing. *Corticosteroids* can help but mechanism of action to reduce fatigue unknown. Consider if patient also has anorexia, nausea/vomiting or bony pain. Dosing 4–8 mg daily

- – Treating symptoms associated with fatigue may improve fatigue (e.g., depression)
- – Complementary medicine approaches generally with limited evidence but may be considered. Modalities include acupuncture, massage and healing touch, hypnosis, mindfulness-based stress reduction, and relaxation/breathing exercises

Psychosocial

- • *Depression* is a part of a broader concept of distress but is distinct; distress in cancer patients is more prevalent. Patients with sadness still feel connected with others, can enjoy happiness, symptoms occur intermittently, and they still feel the will to live
- • Depression can decrease patient's participation in their care, leads to suffering, and potentially prolongs hospital stays
- • Assessment is challenging in cancer care as many symptoms could be due to underlying disease or treatments:

  - – Asking "are you depressed" has 72% sensitivity/83% specificity
  - – Asking about loss of interest has 83% sensitivity/86% specificity
  - – Asking both of above has 91% sensitivity/86% specificity
  - – *Other screening tools:* Visual analogue scale, Beck Depression Inventory Short Form, Hospital Anxiety

and Depression Scale (HADS), Mood Evaluation Questionnaire. and Edinburgh Postnatal Depression Scale:

- Non-pharmacological treatment strategies include multiple types of psychotherapy, massage therapy, and dignity therapy (a type of therapy that involves interviewing patients about their life story and personal history, transcribing the interview and producing it into a document that serves as a legacy for friend and family (Table 7.2)

- Pharmacologic treatment strategies include serotonin-specific reuptake inhibitors (SSRIs) and tricyclic antidepressants (TCAs), or psychostimulants. SSRI therapy may be challenging in those with short prognosis as time to benefit may be 4 weeks or more (Table 7.3)
- *Anxiety:* Persistent anxiety can become excessive, impairing decision-making, worsening symptoms, and interrupting care. Anxiety is more likely to be a pre-existing condition and reactivates during cancer treatment. It exists as four types: situational, psychiatric, organic, and existential

  - Many factors contribute, including uncertainty about disease prognosis, social isolation, medication side effects or withdrawal, and pain. Additional risk factors include advanced cancer and having dependent children
  - *Assessment:* Asking "how anxious have you felt this week" can easily screen for anxiety. Consider using the HADS as well
  - *Non-pharmacological therapies* include psychotherapy, stress management, supportive counseling, education, massage, or music therapy
  - *Pharmacological therapies* include antidepressants, benzodiazepines, and non-benzodiazepine anxiolytics. Some SSRIs can interfere with tamoxifen and would not be recommended (e.g., paroxetine). TCAs may worsen cognitive dysfunction and constipation

TABLE 7.2 Description of psychosocial interventions

Term	Description
Counseling	Generic term used to refer to supportive psychosocial care provided by a qualified professional
Psychoeducation	Provision of information designed to increase knowledge and reduce uncertainty and thereby enhance psychological well-being
Relaxation training	Teaches skills for releasing physical or mental tension using meditative activities, progressive muscle relaxation exercises, or use of guided mental imagery
Problem-solving therapy	Focuses on generating, applying, and evaluating solutions to identified problems
Cognitive behavioral therapy	Focuses on identifying, challenging, and changing maladaptive thoughts and behaviors to reduce negative emotions and promote psychologic adjustment
Interpersonal therapy	Focuses on problems within interpersonal interactions and relationships, emphasizing areas such as grief, role transitions, disputes, or interpersonal deficits to reduce distress and promote psychologic adjustment
Supportive-expressive (psychodynamic) therapy	Focuses on the communication and processing of subjective experience and on the joint creation of meaning within a therapeutic relationship to reduce distress and promote psychologic adjustment (e.g., meaning-centered therapy, dignity therapy, and CALM)

From: (Li et al. 2012). Reprinted with permission. © 2012 American Society of Clinical Oncology. All rights reserved
Abbreviation: *CALM* Managing cancer and living meaningfully

TABLE 7.3 Medications useful for treatment of depression

Drug	Main adverse effects	Major interactions	Considerations/toxicities
SSRIs	Sexual dysfunction, nausea, GI disturbance, sweating, anxiety, headache, sleep disturbance, tremor		Rare akathisia, gastrointestinal bleeding, hyponatremia, bruxism
Citalopram		No significant inhibition of cytochrome P450 enzymes	Generally first-line SSRI choice because well tolerated and few drug-drug interactions
Escitalopram		No significant inhibition of cytochrome P450 enzymes	Generally first-line SSRI choice because well tolerated and few drug-drug interactions
Fluoxetine	No discontinuation symptoms	Strong inhibitor of CYP2D6 and 3A4	Should be avoided in those taking tamoxifen because of 2D6 inhibition
Sertraline		Moderate inhibitor of CYP2D6	

(continued)

Table 7.3 (continued)

Drug	Main adverse effects	Major interactions	Considerations/toxicities
Paroxetine	Discontinuation symptoms common	Strong inhibitor of CYP2D6	Should be avoided in those receiving tamoxifen because of 2D6 inhibition
Fluvoxamine		Moderate inhibitor of CYP2D6, 1A2, and 3A4	
Mixed action			
Venlafaxine (SNRI)	Sexual dysfunction, nausea, insomnia, dry mouth, anxiety, sleep disturbance, headache	No inhibition of cytochrome P450 enzymes	First-line choice for those receiving tamoxifen because of lack of 2D6 inhibition
	Discontinuation symptoms common		Beneficial in reducing hot flashes in women receiving chemotherapy or who have tamoxifen-induced menopause
			May cause elevation of blood pressure at higher doses and should be avoided if risk of arrhythmia

Duloxetine (SNRI)	Similar to venlafaxine, but discontinuation symptoms less common; anorexia	Moderate inhibitor of CYP2D6	Also treatment for diabetic neuropathy and neuropathic pain
			Monitoring required for risk of hepatic failure; contraindicated with significant liver disease
Mirtazapine (NaSSA)	Drowsiness, increased appetite, weight gain. headache, dizziness	Minimal effect on P450 enzymes	Good choice for depressed patients with cancer with loss of appetite and insomnia; less sedating at higher doses
			Available in orally disintegrating tablet
			Minimal effect on sexual functioning

(continued)

Table 7.3 (continued)

Drug	Main adverse effects	Major interactions	Considerations/toxicities
Bupropion (NDM)	Agitation, weight loss, constipation, headache, insomnia, nausea	Strong inhibitor of CYP2D6	Activating properties make it useful in cases of prominent fatigue, hypersomnia, or psychomotor retardation
	Seizure risk (dose dependent)		Minimal effect on sexual functioning
			Also useful as aid in smoking cessation
TCAs	Sedation, postural hypotension, dry mouth, blurred vision, constipation, urinary retention, tachycardia, arrhythmia, delirium	Phenothiazines, some opioids, and SSRIs can increase plasma levels	Also used for neuropathic pain syndromes; poorer tolerability than other antidepressant medications; toxicity in overdose and anticholinergic effects are major drawbacks to their use in psycho-oncology
Amitriptyline			
Nortriptyline			
Desipramine			

Psychostimulants	Insomnia, agitation, euphoria, tremor, anxiety, hypertension, tachycardia, confusion, delirium	May increase levels of SSRIs, TCAs, and some antiepileptics	Stimulating properties have led to use in anergic, depressed patients with cancer with terminal or advanced disease; contraindicated in the presence of significant cardiovascular disease; rapid onset of action (days vs weeks)
Methylphenidate			
Dextroamphetamine			
Modafinil (nonamphetamine)	Adverse effects less frequent		

From: (Li et al. 2012). Reprinted with permission. © 2012 American Society of Clinical Oncology. All rights reserved

Abbreviations: NaSSA noradrenaline and specific serotonergic antidepressant, *NDM* norepinephrine-dopamine modulator, *SNRI* serotonin norepinephrine reuptake inhibitor *SSRI* selective serotonin reuptake inhibitor, *TCA* tricyclic antidepressant

Pain

• Untreated or undertreated pain can impact patient's ability to undergo cancer treatments, to improve functional status, or to die peacefully. Types of pain include *nociceptive* pain (due to ongoing tissue injury that could be either somatic or visceral), *neuropathic* pain (due to peripheral/CNS damage), and *intermittent* pain (due to incident pain)

• As with the other symptoms in this section, pain may occur due to cancer itself, acutely due to treatment, or may persist for months or years following treatment. Management depends on the etiology and phase of cancer care

• While use of opioids is often indicated (and may be underutilized) for those with advanced cancer and those who are being treated palliatively, it is critical to assess for the indication and plan for tapering and/or management for longer-term cancer survivors

• If opioids are used, the WHO cancer pain ladder remains a foundation in pain management (http://www.who.int/cancer/palliative/painladder/en/). Do not start with a sustained-release or transdermal route of opioids to initiate treatment of pain

• General principles for titrating and using opioids:

  – Increase dose based on total daily dose (scheduled + all PRN)

    • For mild pain increase total daily dose by 25%
    • For moderate pain increase total daily dose by 50%
    • For severe pain increase total daily dose by 100% For example, if a patient is on 15 mg MS Contin BID but uses 90 mg of morphine total in 24 h for severe pain, increase the MS Contin to 30 mg BID (a 100% increase)
    • When higher doses of opioids are needed, do not use combination medications (e.g., with acetaminophen) to avoid needing to limit the dose
    • For continuous pain, treat with scheduled opioid with additional doses available for breakthrough pain.

When dose is stable, convert to scheduled long-acting opioid plus immediate release for breakthrough pain. The long-acting mediation should be 50–100% of the total daily dose (scheduled and PRN). Increase extended-release dose if patient needs multiple (i.e., four or more) PRN doses or pain not adequately treated. Breakthrough doses should be 10–20% of the 24 h total of long-acting opioid. Oral breakthrough medications can be dosed up to every 1 h as needed

- Consider rotating to a different opioid if the patient has inadequate response after a fair trial, has intolerable side effects, rapidly develops tolerance, or has refractory pain. Consider palliative care referral if rotation necessary. Use equianalgesic dosing to rotate opioids (Table 7.4)

  – *Steps to convert to different opioid:* Determine total daily dose (scheduled + PRN); calculate equianalgesic dose; dose reduce to allow for incomplete cross tolerance (multiply by 60%) if pain was controlled; divide total amount by # doses per day; adjust the breakthrough accordingly (10–20% daily dose)

- *Steps to rotate to transdermal fentanyl patch:* Calculate total daily dose; determine oral morphine equivalent of that dose; transdermal fentanyl patch dose is 1/2 of oral morphine equivalent
- Fentanyl is lipid soluble and may not be as effective in cachectic patient; transdermal fentanyl patches not recommended for acute pain or for frequent titration. Absorption of fentanyl patch may increase with fever and heat
- Methadone has a very long half-life, and dose escalation should not occur more often than every 5 days. There is no equianalgesic dosing, making rotation difficult. If rotation desired or need to be initiated, recommend palliative care consult
- Tramadol should be avoided in patients on serotonin-specific reuptake inhibitors (SSRIs), on tricyclic antidepressants (TCAs), or with history of seizures

TABLE 7.4 Guide to rotating opioids

Opioid	Parental dose	Oral dose	Dose interval
Morphine	10 mg	30 mg	3–4 h
Morphine sustained release	–	30 mg	Capsules: 12–24 h Tablets: 8–12 h
Oxycodone	–	20 mg	3–4 h
Oxycodone sustained release	–	20 mg	12 h
Hydromorphone	1.5 mg	7.5 mg	
Fentanyl	100 mcg (0.1 mg)	1000 mcg oral transmucosal	0.5–1 h
Fentanyl transdermal	–	–	72 h
Hydrocodone	–	30 mg (dose not recommended)	3–4 h
Codeine	–	200 mg (dose not recommended)	3–4 h

- Morphine should be avoided in renal failure
  - Opioid side effects include:
    - Constipation (see above for management)
    - Nausea (see above for management)
    - Sedation: treat with opioid rotation and psychostimulants
    - Respiratory depression: can occur at any stage of dosing or with rotation; treat with dose reduction or naloxone. If naloxone used, dilute and use as last resort as this could precipitate a pain crisis

- Myoclonus: seen with neurotoxicity; treat with dose reduction, opioid rotation, clonazepam, diazepam, baclofen, valproic acid, and dantrolene
- Delirium
- Sexual dysfunction: due to hypogonadism; check testosterone levels and treat if indicated
- Hyperalgesia: consider adjuvant medication; could also consider ketamine but should refer to pain specialist service if considering
- Pruritus: treat with antihistamines or opioid rotation

  - Adjuvant medications should be considered when pain control is sub-optimal, when side effects/toxicities limit opioid therapy, or when multiple types of pain exist
  - If patient is on clinical trial or immunotherapy, discuss starting corticosteroids with the patient's oncologist prior to initiating treatment
  - Corticosteroids can also be considered for liver capsular stretch pain or bony pain

- *Non-pharmacological interventions:*

  - Radiotherapy can help with bony metastatic pain
  - Nerve blocks
  - Vertebroplasty/kyphoplasty
  - Cognitive behavioral therapy, breathing exercises, relaxation, guided imagery, and hypnosis
  - Massage, heat/cold therapy, acupuncture, and acupressure

Special Populations

- *Individuals living in rural or resource-poor areas* may face challenges in access to specialty services, which increase risk for disparities. Strategies to overcome barriers include:

  - Tele-health/tele-oncology
  - Virtual tumor boards

- Outreach clinics
- Educational and staffing programs for existing rural workforce

- *Pediatric and young adult (YA) patients*

  - May require or prefer input of parents in decision-making process
  - Palliative care should be "family centered" while at the same time respecting the stage of developmental autonomy of the patient
  - Patients should be involved in decision-making process. Status should be reassessed over the course of illness
  - Advance care planning documents should address unique adolescent and YA phase of life concerns (e.g., family planning, young children at home)
  - Important principles of care for this population include providing more clarity with regard to communication of patient wishes in the event of specific life-threatening medical events, respecting a desire for ongoing connection with peer groups, and inquiring specifically about how one would want to be remembered

- *Minority and/or non-English-speaking populations:* Challenges to care can be practical and/or cultural

  - Cultural: Beliefs of health and illness (and role of palliative care) may conflict with those of the healthcare team, or beliefs may not be well understood or well communicated. Strategies to address these concerns include:

    - Assessing how the patient understands his/her illness
    - Addressing religious/spiritual values
    - Determining the patient's desired approach to diagnostic truth telling
    - Understanding how the patient's family is involved in care
    - Negotiating cultural conflicts when they arise

  - Practical: For non-English speakers, use of ad hoc interpreters is common, often family members. Culturally and linguistically appropriate services standards recommend use of professionally trained medical interpreter

- Roles for the interpreter in the clinical encounter should be clarified
- Professional interpreters can help ensure that cultural considerations are taken into account

Additional Resources

- American Academy of Hospice and Palliative Medicine: http://aahpm.org/
- American Society of Clinical Oncology: https://www.asco.org/practice-guidelines/cancer-care-initiatives/palliative-care-oncology
- Choosing Wisely Campaign – http://www.choosingwisely.org/
- Compassion and Choices: https://www.compassionand-choices.org/
- EPEC Modules, an educational resource for healthcare professionals about palliative care – http://bioethics.northwestern.edu/programs/epec/about/index.html
- Fast Facts – https://www.mypcnow.org/
- National Cancer Institute: https://www.cancer.gov/about-cancer/advanced-cancer/care-choices/palliative-care-fact-sheet
- National Comprehensive Cancer Network Palliative Care Clinical Practice Guidelines: www.nccn.org
- National Hospice and Palliative Care Organization: www.nhpco.org
- Oncotalk http://depts.washington.edu/oncotalk/
- Unipac Book Series – http://aahpm.org/self-study/unipacs

References

Ann M. Berger, Amy Pickar Abernethy, Ashley Atkinson, Andrea M. Barsevick, William S. Breitbart, David Cella, Bernadine Cimprich, Charles Cleeland, Mario A. Eisenberger, Carmen P. Escalante, Paul B. Jacobsen, Phyllis Kaldor, Jennifer A. Ligibel,

Barbara A. Murphy, Tracey O'Connor, William F. Pirl, Eve Rodler, Hope S. Rugo, Jay Thomas, Lynne I. Wagner, (2010) Cancer-Related Fatigue. Journal of the National Comprehensive Cancer Network 8 (8):904–31.

Bernacki RE, Block SD, for the American College of Physicians High Value Care Task Force. Communication About Serious Illness Care Goals. A Review and Synthesis of Best Practices. JAMA Intern Med. 2014;174(12):1994–2003.

Bruera E, Kuehn N, Miller MJ, Selmser P. The Edmonton Symptom Assessment System (ESAS): a simple method for the assessment of palliative care patients. J Palliat Care. 1991;7:6–9.

Chochinov HM, Hack T, Hassard T, Kristjanson LJ, McClement S, Harlos M. Dignity therapy: a novel psychotherapeutic intervention for patients near the end of life. J Clin Oncol. 2005;23(24): 5520–5.

Current Procedural Terminology (CPT) Professional. Chicago, Il: American Medical Association; 2016.

Denlinger CS, Ligibel JA, Are M, Baker KS, Demark-Wahnefried W, Friedman DL, et al. Survivorship: fatigue, version 1.2014. J Natl Compr Cancer Netw. 2014;12(6):876–87.

Dumanovsky T, Augustin R, Rogers M, Lettang K, Meier DE, Morrison RS. The growth of palliative care in U.S. hospitals: a status report. J Palliat Med. 2016;19(1):8–15.

Fischer SM, Gozansky WS, Sauaia A, Min SJ, Kutner JS, Kramer A. A practical tool to identify patients who may benefit from a palliative approach: the CARING criteria. J Pain Symptom Manage. 2006;31(4):285–92.

Glare PA, Chow K. Validation of a simple screening tool for identifying unmet palliative care needs in patients with cancer. J Oncol Pract. 2015;11(1):e81–6.

Houben CHM, Spruit MA, Groenen MTJ, Wouters EFM, Janssen DJA. Efficacy of advance care planning: a systematic review and meta-analysis. J Am Med Dir Assoc. 2014;15(7):477–89.

Jennings AL, Davies AN, Higgins JP, Broadley K. Opioids for the palliation of breathlessness in terminal illness. Cochrane Database Syst Rev. 2001; (4):CD002066.

Johnson MJ, Hui D, Currow DC. Opioids, exertion, and dyspnea: a review of the evidence. Am J Hospice Palliat Med. 2016;33(2):194–200.

Jones CA, Acevedo J, Bull J, Kamal AH. Top 10 tips for using advance care planning codes in palliative medicine and beyond. J Palliat Med. 2016;19(12):1249–53.

Kamal AH, Maguire JM, Wheeler JL, Currow DC, Abernethy AP. Dyspnea review for the palliative care professional: assessment, burdens, and etiologies. J Palliat Med. 2011;14(10): 1167–72.

Kamal AH, Maguire JM, Wheeler JL, Currow DC, Abernethy AP. Dyspnea review for the palliative care professional: treatment goals and therapeutic options. J Palliat Med. 2012;15(1):106–14.

Klaschik E, Nauck F, Ostgathe C. Constipation—modern laxative therapy. Support Care Cancer. 2003;11(11):679–85.

Li M, Fitzgerald P, Rodin G. Evidence-based treatment of depression in patients with cancer. J Clin Oncol. 2012;30(11):1187–96.

Librach SL, Bouvette M, De Angelis C, Farley J, Oneschuk D, Pereira JL, et al. Consensus recommendations for the management of constipation in patients with advanced, progressive illness. J Pain Symptom Manage. 2010;40(5):761–73.

Mitchell AJ. Are one or two simple questions sufficient to detect depression in cancer and palliative care? A Bayesian meta-analysis. Br J Cancer. 2008;98(12):1934–43.

Moss AH, Lu nney JR, Culp S, Auber M, Kurian S, Rogers J, et al. Prognostic significance of the "surprise" question in cancer patients. J Palliat Med. 2010;13(7):837–40.

Nalamachu SR, Pergolizzi J, Taylor R, Slatkin NE, Barrett AC, Yu J, et al. Efficacy and tolerability of subcutaneous methylnaltrexone in patients with advanced illness and opioid-induced constipation: a responder analysis of 2 randomized, placebo-controlled trials. Pain Pract. 2015;15(6):564–71.

National Consensus Project for Quality Palliative Care. Clinical practice guidelines for quality palliative care. 4th ed. 2018. National Consensus Project for Quality Palliative Care. The National Coalition for Hospice and Palliative Care. https://www.nationalcoalitionhpc.org/ncp-guidelines-2018/.

National Palliative Care Registry at the Center to Advance Palliative Care. Growth of Palliative Care in US Hospitals 2016 Snapshot (2000–2015). New York: Center to Advance Palliative Care. 2016. https://registry.capc.org/metrics-resources/registry-publications/.

Partain DK, Ingram C, Strand JJ. Providing appropriate end-of-life care to religious and ethnic minorities. Mayo Clin Proceed. 2017;92(1):147–52.

Schulz R, Beach SR. Caregiving as a risk factor for mortality: the Caregiver Health Effects study. JAMA. 1999;282(23):2215–9.

Sepúlveda C, Marlin A, Yoshida T, Ullrich A. Palliative care: the World Health Organization's global perspective. J Pain Sympt Manage. 2002;24(2):91–6.

Spence RA, Blanke CD, Keating TJ, Taylor LP. Responding to patient requests for hastened death: physician aid in dying and the clinical oncologist. J Oncol Pract. 2017;13(10):693–9.

Sulmasy DP, Finlay I, Fitzgerald F, Foley K, Payne R, Siegler M. Physician-assisted suicide: why neutrality by organized medicine is neither neutral nor appropriate. J Gen Intern Med. 2018 May 2.

Wiencek C, Coyne P. Palliative Care Delivery Models. Seminars in Oncology Nursing. 2014;30(4):227–233.

World Health Organization. Definition of palliative care. http://www.who.int/cancer/palliative/definition/en/. Accessed 27 May 2018.

Youngwerth J, Min S-j, Statland B, Allyn R, Fischer S. Caring about prognosis: a validation study of the caring criteria to identify hospitalized patients at high risk for death at 1 year. J Hosp Med. 2013;8(12):696–701.

Index

© Springer Nature Switzerland AG 2019
L. Nekhlyudov et al. (eds.), *Caring for Patients Across the Cancer Care Continuum*,
https://doi.org/10.1007/978-3-030-01896-2